C000185415

1

2

3

steps

to

fertility

1

2

3
steps
to
fertility

Marina Nicholas

with Dr. Mohammed Taranissi

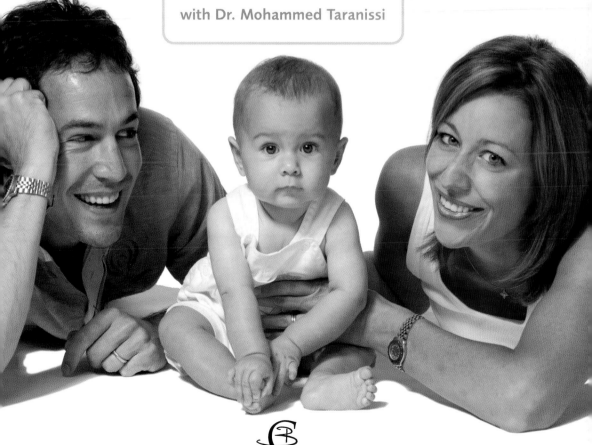

CARROLL & BROWN PUBLISHERS LIMITED

To Simon and Bruno

First published in 2006 in the United Kingdom by

Carroll & Brown Publishers Limited
20 Lonsdale Road
London NW6 6RD

Text © Marina Nicholas 2006
Illustrations and compilation © Carroll & Brown Limited 2006

A CIP catalogue record for this book is available from
the British Library.

ISBN 1-904760-25-2

10987654321

The moral right of Marina Nicholas to be identified as the author
of this work has been asserted in accordance with the Copyright,
Designs and Patents Act of 1988.

All rights reserved. No part of this publication may be
reproduced in any material form (including photocopying or
storing it in any medium by electronic means and whether or not
transiently or incidentally to some other use of this publication)
without the written permission of the copyright owner, except in
accordance with the provisions of the Copyright, Designs and
Patents Act of 1988 or under the terms of a licence issued by the
Copyright Licensing Agency, 90 Tottenham Court Road, London
W1P 9HE. Applications for the copyright owner's written
permission to reproduce any part of this publication should be
addressed to the publisher.

Reproduced by RALI, Bilbao, Spain
Printed and bound in Italy by MS Printing

contents

Foreword 6   Introduction 8

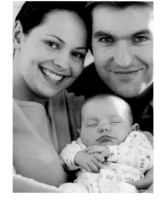

Step 1

Understand your body
10 – 65

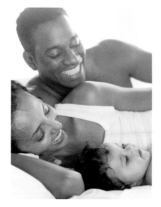

Step 2

Complete
the tests
66 – 81

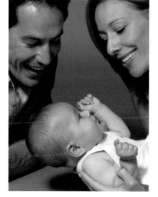

Step 3

Choose a treatment
82 – 145

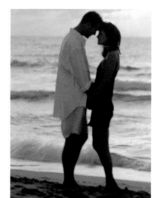

Emotional
issues
146 – 154

References 155
Useful addresses 157
Index 158
Acknowledgments 160

Foreword

In 1996, just after I got married, I discovered I had been silently suffering with endometriosis. The condition was uncovered during an internal investigation, which showed adhesions around my fallopian tubes and ovaries. The consultant told me that if I hadn't yet considered starting a family I should do so soon as the damage might make it difficult to have a baby naturally. This news came as a bolt out of the blue. My husband, Simon, and I had discussed having a family in the future; suddenly the decision was made. We had to start trying straight away.

My story is like that of thousands of other women in the world who are faced with the news that having a baby may not be as straightforward as they initially thought. From that day I embarked on a journey to understand every facet of infertility – why it happens and how conventional and complementary therapies can assist women in increasing their chances of having a baby.

My interest in the human body started at a young age and led me to complete a BSC (Hons) in Human Biological Sciences at Loughborough University. I remember my entrance interview very well. The tutor asked me why I wished to study human biology. My answer was simple and stands true to this day 'The human body is amazing – it gives us the miracle of life'. Since then, reading about the human body has been my hobby especially with the new and exciting Eastern therapies becoming more widely available in the West. Even today the most sophisticated modern technology of creating a test tube baby (IVF) only achieves an average success rate of 25 percent in the UK. Seventy-five percent of couples walk away without any success, and are only offered a glimmer of hope for the next time. Currently, one in five couples in the UK have some kind of infertility problem. There is a need to continually learn more about the human body, how it functions and what we can do to help maximise the chance of having a healthy baby.

Over the last seven years, Simon and I have learnt a lot about the medical profession, the field of infertility and, above all, about each other. We have experienced two natural pregnancies, five IVF attempts, two ectopic pregnancies, one miscarriage, one near-death experience and the ultimate joy of bringing baby Bruno into this world. It has been one hell of a ride! I could never have anticipated this happening 10 years ago but we came through it by taking it one step at a time. We feel like we have climbed to the top of Mount Everest and are now enjoying the wonderful view, the joy of parenthood.

It is because our situation is like that of many other couples faced with infertility, that we wish to share our experiences and knowledge, so they, too, can have the immense pleasure of bringing a baby into this world.

My diagnosis seven years ago led me to study the conventional, the unconventional, the scientific and the spiritual practices that exist to improve the chances of conception. If, seven years ago, I had been able to read a book that gave me a complete overview of these practices, I would have been better able to make the right decisions. As it happened, I had to read many books, research the Internet, and try out each and every treatment myself to find the right one for Simon and me.

This book was written to give you the head start I wish I had had. It will help you understand what you can do to maximise your chances of conceiving a baby. We are all different people in different situations and there is no 'one size fits all' in matters of infertility treatment. You may be more comfortable starting off looking at your nutrition and lifestyle rather than starting on fertility drugs straight away. Or you may prefer to look at any psychological barriers you may have that might interfere with you having a baby instead of stimulating your ovaries through acupuncture. Or maybe you want to try the least expensive and invasive options before worrying about how you will finance other treatments.

This book will give you hope while you find the right approach for you and your partner. There are no guarantees that you will conceive a baby but by reading this book you will be more open to all the treatments and be better informed to progress on your journey. This book aims to combine conventional and complementary approaches to achieve conception – the dream!

Wishing you much success!

Maxine Nicholas

Introduction

Why the 3 steps?

Recently there has been an enormous amount of literature written on the field of infertility. Even TV documentaries and chat shows are featuring women telling their heartfelt stories as people are becoming more aware of the rise of infertility cases in the UK.

If you have been unsuccessful in conceiving a baby it is difficult to know where to start. This is the problem I faced seven years ago. Gynaecologists, midwives and naturopaths write most of the books on infertility but they approach infertility from the perspective of how to treat a couple. No books have been written by someone with infertility who has tried to make sense of it all!

It is difficult to get inside the minds of a couple faced with infertility, to know what they expect, how they feel and how they will react. Guilt, frustration, depression, anxiety, failure, longing, jealousy, denial, anger and loneliness are but a few of the emotions that infertile couples experience at some point. How can the 'experts' begin to understand couples like us, they must be thinking.

Over the years I have collected piles of information about infertility and I decided it was time to write about infertility from an infertile couple's perspective. I would interpret the medical information and aim to provide the right amount of sympathy, encouragement and support to answer the question all infertile couples desperately want answered – what can I do to increase my chances of having a baby? The idea for this book was born.

When collating all my research, it became apparent that it fell naturally into three piles – information about the body and the causes of infertility, the process of testing male and female fertility and, finally, the largest and most diverse pile, all the treatment options, complementary and conventional.

I have personally tried all the treatments and would not include them in this book if I did not feel each one had its merits. It is up to you to choose the one(s) with which one you feel comfortable. Doctors are quick to recommend drug-induced treatments, often justly so, but for some couples it may be their last choice. So what are the three steps?

step 1 **Gain a full understanding of the male and female body, the cycles involved in conception and the reasons for infertility.**

- What are the main causes?
- How does age affect fertility?
- Can my lifestyle affect my fertility?
- What psychological factors affect fertility?
- Can weight affect my fertility?
- What can go wrong?
- Am I ready for pregnancy?
- Complete a lifestyle questionnaire to reveal potential problem areas.

step 2 **Find out what the problem is by completing the necessary fertility tests at the appropriate time.**

- What are the male and female tests for infertility?
- How can I establish if my body had the right vitamins and minerals for conception?
- Am I full of toxins?

step 3 **Choose the complementary or conventional treatment that will improve your chances of having a baby.**

- How can changing my diet and lifestyle improve my fertility?
- Which vitamins and minerals are essential for conception?
- What is the preconception diet?
- Complete a three-month preconception plan.
- Can hypnotherapy, reflexology, acupuncture or herbal medicine help me? How?
- How do I choose a clinic?
- How do I interpret a clinic's published information?
- What drug-induced treatments are available?
- What is the process of IVF?
- Are there other options? Adoption? Surrogacy?

My aim is to help as many couples as possible to increase their chances of having a baby. If you follow the three steps to fertility, you and your partner will be on the right path. This book was written by someone who completed the uphill struggle and has you in mind every step of the way.

step 1

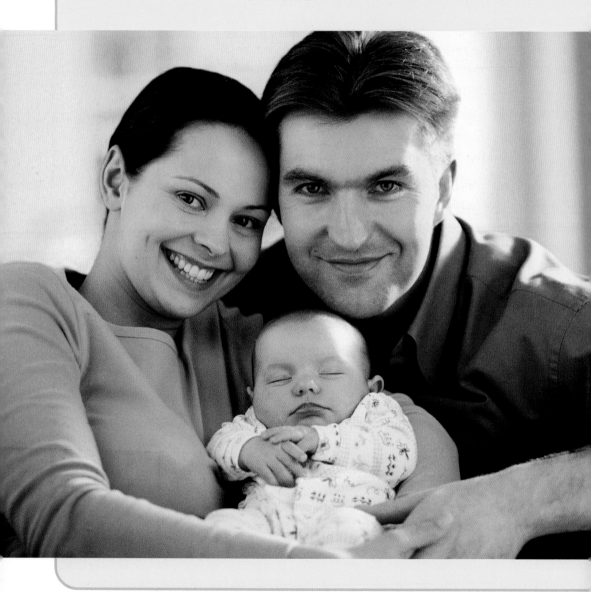

Understand your body

the reproductive system, the cycles involved in conception and the causes of infertility

The first step towards fertility is to understand how your body works. It sounds simple but there are hundreds of processes that need to come into play in order for a sperm and egg to combine and create a baby.

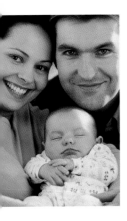

Having read many infertility books over the years I have seen my fair share of medical terms, explanations, diagrams and charts. Often, I confess, I skipped past the boring medical information and jumped straight to the sections about my problem and how it could be treated. With hindsight, I was too impatient and should have ploughed through all the information before making the 'wrong' assumption. I believed endometriosis was the sole cause of my infertility but it later became apparent that my fallopian tubes were also a contributing factor. I might have realised this sooner if I had read the breadth of information available on symptoms and causes, rather than becoming totally focussed on the one discovered issue.

With that in mind I have tried to keep this chapter informative – with sufficient medical terms to empower you – but also with anecdotal evidence and stories that should keep you motivated to read the chapter in its entirety. If I have failed, you will flick through to chapter 3 and may become confused like I did!

My aim in this chapter is to
- give you essential background information;
- help you understand medical professionals and speak their language;
- assist you in understanding medical terminology;
- arm you with the right questions to ask about your problem, and finally …
- give you and your partner confidence as you embark on your journey of discovery.

Many couples get pregnant after having sex for the first time, while others may try to conceive for years. So why is it more difficult for some people? It is easy to assume that getting pregnant is relatively simple, yet in order for conception to take place, many biological processes have to come together at exactly the right time. The man needs to produce robust sperm and the woman healthy eggs; the cervical mucus needs to be supportive and abundant so that the sperm can travel up through the cervical canal to the uterus and fallopian tubes; the fallopian tubes need to be open and accessible so that the sperm can reach the egg; the sperm has to be able to fertilise the egg when they make contact; the

fertilised egg (the embryo) has to be able to implant in the woman's uterus; and, finally, both the embryo and the woman's uterine environment need to be healthy and strong for the baby to grow to full term. If any one of these processes is impaired or damaged in any way, infertility can result. Moreover, aging, a history of pelvic inflammatory disease, and certain lifestyle behaviours can also make a woman infertile.

Infertility currently affects one in five couples and is predicted to increase to one in three couples within the next five years.

By having a full understanding of the mechanics of the male and female reproductive system, you and your partner will increase your chances of conceiving at the right time in the right environment.

The female reproductive system

The female organs

First let's look at the main components of the female reproductive system – the ovaries, the fallopian tubes and uterus.

The ovaries

About the size of walnuts, the ovaries are located just below the fallopian tubes on each side of the uterus. The ovaries contain a woman's egg supply and it is the site where the egg will develop each month in fluid-filled sacs called follicles. The ovaries also produce the female sex hormones, oestrogen and progesterone. A woman is born with an abundant supply of several million eggs, which over time diminishes to approximately 400,000 by the time she reaches puberty. The rate of loss continues until the menopause starts at about the age of fifty. Each month after puberty, many of the unripened eggs will start the developmental process but usually only one is released during ovulation. After the egg is released from the ovary it is picked up by the fallopian tube.

Fallopian tubes

The fallopian tubes extend from the uterus up around the ovaries. They are responsible for collecting the newly released egg, providing nutrients and movement for it and sustaining a healthy environment for fertilisation. Fimbriae, the fan-like fingers at the ends of the tubes, draw the released egg into the uterus. The tubes produce a series of muscular contractions that push the egg down; if the egg meets sperm coming up the tube, fertilisation can take place. Once fertilisation occurs, the resulting embryo travels the remaining length of the fallopian tube to the uterus (this may take a few days). If the fallopian tubes are damaged (from tubal disease, for example, see pages 20–23), the embryo will be unable to travel and will implant into the side of the fallopian tube. This is called an ectopic pregnancy. An ectopic pregnancy is a potentially life-threatening situation and surgical intervention is needed to remove the embryo and usually the fallopian tube in which it has implanted.

The uterus

Also called the womb, the uterus is a hollow, pear-shaped organ located at the base of the pelvic cavity. It protects, develops and nourishes the fetus until birth. At its lower end, a narrow opening called the cervix serves as a passageway for menstrual blood and for giving birth. The uterine lining, known as the endometrium, builds up during the luteal phase of the menstrual cycle (see page 14) in anticipation of receiving an embryo from the fallopian tube. If a pregnancy doesn't occur, it is then shed as menstrual blood during menstruation.

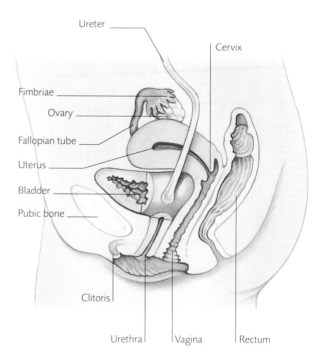

Ureter

Cervix

Fimbriae

Ovary

Fallopian tube

Uterus

Bladder

Pubic bone

Clitoris

Urethra

Vagina

Rectum

The menstrual cycle

A woman's reproductive system undergoes several changes throughout the menstrual cycle in preparation for fertilisation. These are known as:

- Follicular phase
- Ovulation
- Luteal phase

To maximise your chances of conception, it is key that you can interpret the body changes occurring and become an expert of your menstrual cycle. Most books and articles refer to the menstrual cycle typically lasting 28 days; however, many women deviate from the norm –

having cycles of 21 to 40 days – and still successfully conceive. A woman who menstruates for three days, for example, may then have a short first stage, which means she may ovulate as early as day 11. Her menstrual cycle would therefore be about 24 days long, yet she can still conceive if she is aware of when ovulation took place.

Follicular phase

Measured from the first day of the period (bleeding normally occurs for 3 to 7 days), this phase lasts for about the first 14 to 15 days of the cycle. While the uterus sheds its lining, the pituitary gland in the brain releases a hormone called FSH (follicle stimulating hormone). FSH

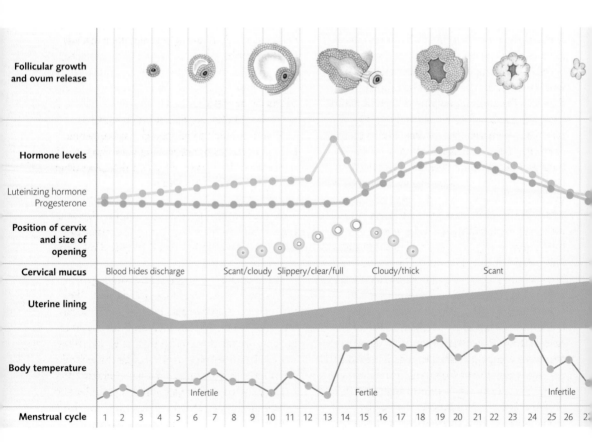

CHARTING THE MENSTRUAL CYCLE CHANGES
Over the course of each monthly cycle, there are changes to hormone levels, the appearance of cervical mucus and the uterine lining, and in body temperature that coincide with the growth,

development and release of an ovum. Being aware of these changes – and what they mean as regards your fertile and infertile days – can help you increase your chances of becoming pregnant.

stimulates the ovaries to mature some of their egg-containing follicles. About 10 to 20 follicles develop but only one will fully mature. As they mature, the follicles produce increasingly high levels of oestrogen that cause the uterine lining to thicken in preparation for a fertilised egg. There is no definite way of knowing from day one of your cycle exactly when ovulation will take place, which is why interpreting your body signs is important when looking at the best time to conceive.

Ovulation

Once the oestrogen from the follicles reaches a certain level, the pituitary gland releases a hormone called LH (luteinising hormone). This causes the most mature follicle to burst open and release its egg into the fallopian tube. The egg is released from the ovary 24 to 36 hours after this LH surge. This is ovulation.

During this time, if a sperm penetrates the egg, fertilisation occurs and an embryo begins to develop. The most fertile time is considered to span the few days before ovulation up to a few days after ovulation. Sperm can survive up to seven days in a woman's body, though the average is a few days. Having sexual intercourse a few days prior to ovulation may mean that the sperm are still alive when the egg is released. The egg can survive for up to 24 hours following ovulation, which is why having sexual intercourse over this period is the key to success. A few days after ovulation, the body enters the luteal phase and is no longer considered fertile.

Luteal phase

Once the egg has been released, the empty follicle it leaves behind forms into a small cyst known as the corpus luteum, which produces progesterone. This causes the lining of the womb to secrete nourishing fluids and oestrogen. Under the influence of progesterone, the uterine wall thickens in preparation to accept an impregnated egg at about day 20. If the egg is not fertilised, the corpus luteum degenerates, oestrogen and progesterone levels fall and the uterine wall breaks down and is shed (menstruation). The pituitary gland detects the falling oestrogen levels and produces FSH, thus beginning a new cycle.

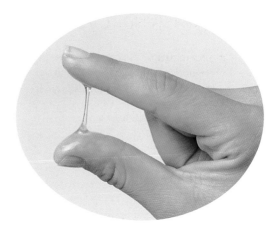

CERVICAL MUCUS
Changes in the texture and appearance of the mucus can help to determine fertile periods. You produce mucus that is clear, stretchy and slippery when you are most fertile.

Signs of ovulation

A number of changes take place to signal ovulation is about to happen or has happened. For the purposes of maximising your chances of conception, focus your efforts on detecting when ovulation is about to happen.

About to happen The most common sign is a change in the cervical mucus as the menstrual cycle progresses. It is a quick, easy and reliable indication of ovulation.

At the beginning of your cycle, oestrogen levels are low and little mucus is present. The dryness means you are relatively infertile at this stage. As your cycle advances, mucus begins to increase in quantity and takes on a white, milky or cloudy consistency, which suggests the fertile period is approaching. Just before ovulation, the mucus changes to become slippery, stretchy and clear – like raw egg white. This is the most fertile period of your cycle. The slippery mucus facilitates the movement of sperm towards an egg in the fallopian tube.

After ovulation, the mucus changes consistency again to a thicker, cloudier, acidic mucus. Typically, four days after the last 'egg-white mucus', the infertile phase begins.

15

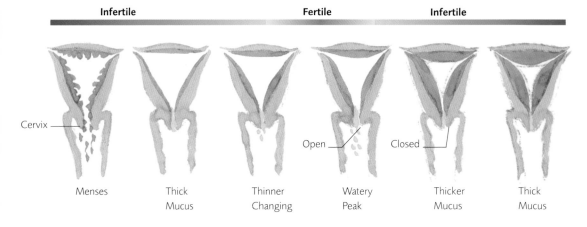

| Infertile | | | Fertile | Infertile | |

Cervix

Open — Closed —

| Menses | Thick Mucus | Thinner Changing | Watery Peak | Thicker Mucus | Thick Mucus |

Has happened Taking your basal body temperature each morning over a few months will help you identify if you ovulate on a regular basis. It is important to know this when considering treatment options. Many women have anovulatory cycles (do not ovulate) and are not aware of it. Typically the temperature is a little below the recognised figure of 37°C (98.6°F). A woman's early morning temperature is lower during the first half of her menstrual cycle by a fraction of a degree. The change in the temperature record from low to high occurs at the time of ovulation. It then shows a drop of 0.1°C to 0.2°C (0.2°F to 0.4°F) at the time of ovulation followed the next day by a rise to the level above that previously recorded (see below).

Tracking your basal body temperature does not tell you when you are fertile or about to ovulate, it tells you only that you have (or may not have) ovulated. Women are most fertile the few days before the peak temperature and once the temperature has remained high for three days, they are least fertile.

CHANGES TO THE CERVIX
Over the course of your cycle, the mucus discharge will change in colour, consistency and amount. Being aware of these changes and what they mean can help you become pregnant (see page 14).

Some women experience a slight twinge in the lower back at the time of ovulation called mittelschmerz (middle pain). Some may also have a discharge that is pinkish in colour at this time or a tingling sensation in the breasts. These bodily signs are minor indicators of ovulation having occurred.

CHANGES IN TEMPERATURE
Another important sign of fertility is the slight changes in temperature that can be recorded on special thermometers.

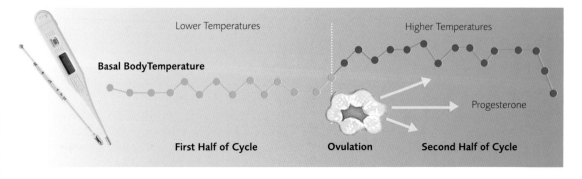

Lower Temperatures — Higher Temperatures

Basal Body Temperature

Progesterone

First Half of Cycle — **Ovulation** — **Second Half of Cycle**

The male reproductive system

The male organs

The male reproductive system consists of external and internal structures whose main function is to produce, maintain and transport sperm and semen, discharge sperm within the female reproductive tract and produce and secrete male sex hormones

The external organs

The penis is the male organ for sexual intercourse. At its tip is the opening of the urethra, which transports semen and urine. During sexual intercourse, muscular contractions within the penis will ejaculate the semen into a woman's vagina.

The scrotum is the pouch of skin behind the penis containing the testicles. It is responsible for temperature regulation – sperm development requires a cooler temperature than that of the body.

The internal organs

Located within the scrotum are two olive-sized testicles or testes. They are responsible for producing testosterone, the male sex hormone, and generating sperm. Sperm cells are produced in the mass of coiled tubes called seminiferous tubules within the testes – in a process called spermatogenesis.

The epididymis is the long coiled tube within the testes which stores the sperm cells and transfers mature ones into the vas deferens.

A long muscular tube, the vas deferens carries the mature sperm to the urethra in preparation for ejaculation. The urethra is the tube that carries urine from the bladder, and semen during sexual intercourse, to outside the body. The prostate gland is located near and empties into the urethra. It contains fluids that nourish the sperm and provides additional fluid to the ejaculate.

Sperm development

The entire male reproductive system is dependent on hormones released by the pituitary gland in the brain. The primary reproductive hormones in males and females are similar. In the males, FSH (follicle-stimulating hormone) is necessary for sperm production (spermatogenesis), LH (luteinizing hormone) stimulates the production of testosterone and testosterone is responsible for the development of male characteristics, sexual arousal and sperm maturation. The testicles typically produce 50,000 new sperm every minute of every day beginning at puberty until a man is 70 years old or older.

Sperm development takes place in the seminiferous tubules of the testes. Cell division produces mature sperm cells that contain one-

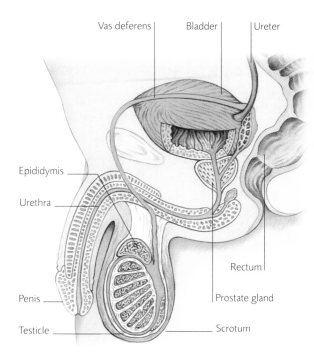

Vas deferens | Bladder | Ureter

Epididymis

Urethra

Rectum

Penis

Prostate gland

Testicle

Scrotum

half of a man's genetic code – 23 chromosomes. Approximately five cycles, or 72 days, are needed to produce one mature sperm. This is equivalent to about three months. Later I discuss the benefits of starting a preconception plan three months before trying to conceive (see page 94). This plan focuses on the benefits of a healthy, nutritious diet while avoiding toxins like alcohol, caffeine and cigarettes, all of which have detrimental effects on the structure of the sperm. One of the key reasons for the three-month time span is to enable your body to eliminate the negative influences any previous lifestyle may have caused and start afresh, essentially with a new batch of sperm.

Sperm are microscopic, naked to the human eye. Each sperm cell consists of a head (acrosome), which carries the genetic make-up (23 chromosomes), a midportion, the energy powerhouse, and a tail (flagella) allowing the sperm to swim and penetrate the egg.

The sperm leave the tubules when almost mature and move along the fine tubes of the epididymis to complete their maturation into a fully mobile healthy sperm. During the final part of their journey, the sperm cells will move into the vas deferens, wait for the muscular contractions associated with sexual arousal, and combine with fluid from the prostate gland before ejaculating through the urethra.

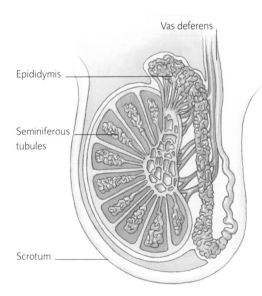

Acrosome
cap

Head
containing
chromosomes

Tail

Midportion

Vas deferens

Epididymis

Seminiferous
tubules

Scrotum

SPERM FACTORY
The many tiny convoluted tubes, known as the seminiferous tubules, inside the testicles are responsible for manufacturing sperm.

Size matters

- One sperm takes about 72 days to develop

- The coiled tubes of the epididymis are 5.4 m (18ft) long

- Ejaculate contains up to 300 million sperm, only one million reach the cervix, 200 reach the fallopian tube and one fertilises an egg

- Two-thirds of a man's sexual system is inside his body, not on the outside

- Each testis has about 250 separate chambers

- Sperm production occurs only at about four degrees below normal body temperature. A higher temperature not only prevents sperm production, but kills sperm in storage

- Semen typically has 2 percent sperm and 98 percent fluid

Fertilisation and implantation

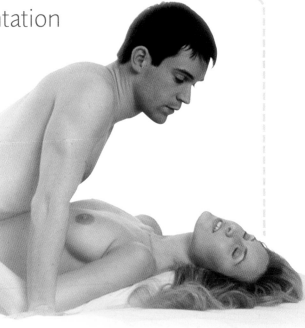

During sexual intercourse the man will ejaculate, releasing between 60 to 150 million sperm into the woman's vagina. The sperm enter the uterus within ten minutes having swum at a speed of 2 to 3 millimetres per minute. The healthy sperm usually reach the egg in the fallopian tube within two hours.

To give you and your partner the best chance of fertilisation, do not rush to get up; relax, watch TV or have a good old chat in bed. The body needs some time to get on with the job at hand!

If the egg successfully fertilises, it will implant in the surface of the uterus about 8 days later – it may take a whole week to travel down the fallopian tube to the uterus! It is important not to do any strenuous activity during this week – the egg may have fertilised but not implanted yet. It is easy to assume that once you have found your fertile period and had sexual intercourse that is it. I personally believe the week following ovulation, when the fertilised egg is still on its travels to the uterus, is just as important. Keep activities light; certainly no running on the treadmill!

The first cell division takes place within 12 hours of fertilisation. Four days after fertilisation, the egg has grown to the size of a blackberry and is ready for implantation. The protective shell surrounding the egg, now known as a blastocyst, is shed to allow it to burrow into the uterine wall. Successful implantation has the effect of releasing hCG (Human Chorionic Gonadotrophin) to maintain the pregnancy – hCG is the hormone detected by pregnancy tests. Progesterone and oestrogen levels continue to rise for up to three months after implantation to ensure the continuation of the pregnancy, at which time the placenta takes over.

MARINA'S STORY

Simon and I realised how important this stage was and we would try all sorts of weird and wonderful things to get his sperm and my egg to meet. After lovemaking, I would lie in bed with my legs up against the wall for about 20 minutes thinking I was helping the little sperm swim with gravity; Simon would sometimes jiggle my hips from side to side; I even tried head stands, except my head would hurt after a few minutes! Did it work? Who knows … But we had a laugh trying and it distracted us from the mechanical aspects of our lovemaking that had become very familiar since trying to conceive. Let's face it: most of us will try anything if we think it will help!

Reasons for infertility

Infertility is defined by the Department of Health as failure to conceive after one year of unprotected sex. Infertility affects both men and women.

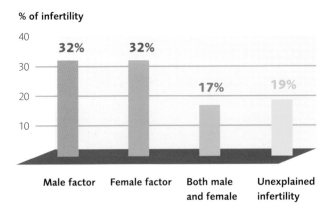

% of infertility

CAUSES OF INFERTILITY BY SEX
Research carried out in 2003 by the Human Fertilisation and Embryology Authority (HFEA) showed that 32 percent of the causes of infertility can be attributed to female problems, 32 percent to male problems, 17 percent to a combination both. The remaining 19 percent falls into a category called unexplained infertility, where a specific problem could not be found in either the man or the woman.

FEMALE FACTORS

Tubal disease and ovulation problems are the two most common causes of infertility in women, accounting for over 70 percent of cases. In five percent of cases a woman has more than one problem causing her infertility.

Tubal disease involves structural or functional damage to one or both fallopian tubes, making it difficult for the sperm to fertilise the egg or the embryo to travel to the uterus.

Ovulatory problems arise when the ovaries do not produce eggs normally. This may be prompted by a number of causes including stress, weight change, failure to ovulate regularly, Polycystic Ovary Syndrome (PCOS) or disorders of the pituitary gland.

Endometriosis, a condition in which the lining of the uterus is found in abnormal locations, may affect the normal functioning of body tissues.

Uterine problems, involving a structural or functional disorder of the uterus, account for 0.3 percent of cases

Other causes include chromosomal abnormalities, serious illness, cancer treatment, etc., account for three percent of cases while multiple factors, where there is more than one reason for infertility, account for five percent. In this chapter we will look at each category in greater detail to understand how these problems affect the reproductive organs and affect fertility.

Tubal disease

This is any problem that affects the fallopian tubes and the organs or tissue surrounding them. The fallopian tube is the actual site of fertilisation and early embryo development. It is a complex structure in which a number of delicate processes come together to aid conception and delivery of the embryo to the womb for implantation. Many of the conditions interfere with the ability of the sperm to reach the egg following ovulation.

The possible causes of tubal problems include endometriosis, inflammation and scarring from pelvic or abdominal surgery such as surgery to remove the appendix in childhood, or previous PID (pelvic inflammatory disease).

Infections like chlamydia and gonorrhea ascend from the uterus to the fallopian tube causing damage to the structure of the tube and the tiny hairs (cilia) lining it. One result of damaged cilia is an ectopic pregnancy, where the embryo grows attached to the wall of the tube itself. Ectopic pregnancy can result in rupturing of the tube, internal bleeding and further tubal damage as the embryo begins to grow in size. Women with a history of PID are six to 10 times more likely to have an ectopic pregnancy compared to women with no previous history.

What is PID (pelvic inflammatory disease)?
This is severe inflammation that results when vaginal and cervical infections spread into the uterus, fallopian tubes, ovaries and surrounding tissues. PID is said to be on the rise in Europe and the United States. This is due to the fact that the average age of a person's first sexual encounter continues to get younger and the time between this encounter and marriage has lengthened, meaning that more people are experimenting with changing partners and increasing their ability to acquire and pass on infections.

A woman or man can experience one episode of PID or it can be a persistent condition that can cause severe damage if left untreated. Up to 40 percent of untreated lower genital tract infections progress to a more serious PID. The two most common genital tract infections are the

Few couples are totally infertile; most are 'subfertile' – that is, they have problems that make conceiving difficult, if not highly unlikely, without medical help. It is estimated that 80 million people worldwide have problems conceiving.

bacterium chlamydia trachomatis (chlamydia) and bacterium neisseria gonorrhoea (gonorrhoea). In total there are about 20 sexually transmitted diseases (STDs) that can cause problems if left untreated so it is wise to have a check up to ensure you and your partner are not infected prior to trying for a baby.

So how do these bacteria access the upper reproductive tract? During most of a woman's menstrual cycle, the cervical mucus at the opening of the cervix is thick and acts like a plug, keeping sperm and bacteria from entering the uterus. The plug dissipates during ovulation and menstruation, making it easier for bacteria to enter the uterus and upper reproductive tract. Also during menstruation, many women experience retrograde menstruation. This backward flow can carry microorganisms as it moves back from the uterus to the fallopian tubes. Once the infection takes root, the body responds to combat the infection by filling the

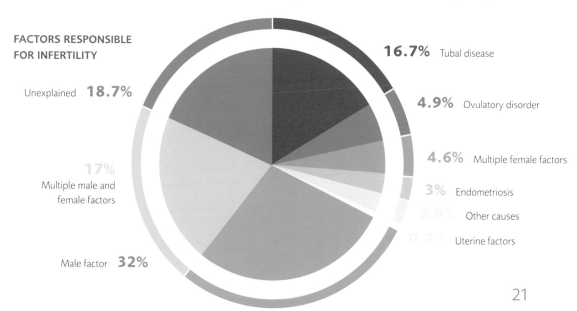

FACTORS RESPONSIBLE FOR INFERTILITY

Unexplained **18.7%**

16.7% Tubal disease

4.9% Ovulatory disorder

4.6% Multiple female factors

17%
Multiple male and female factors

3% Endometriosis

2.9% Other causes

0.3% Uterine factors

Male factor **32%**

The most common STDs affecting fertility

Infection	Symptoms	Treatment/and if left untreated
Chlamydia is the most common STD in the UK, caused by the bacterium chlamydia trachomatis. It is estimated that 1 in 10 adolescents are infected.	25 percent of infected people may have a slight white discharge or stinging on passing urine. Often called the 'silent' disease as 75 percent of women and 50 percent of men have no symptoms. In women: constant lower abdominal pain, mild, milky or yellow discharge, nausea or fever, spotting between periods, pain during intercourse. In men: may have urinary symptoms e.g. burning sensation, discomfort on passing urine.	Course of antibiotics. It is important to treat both partners so the risk of reinfection is reduced. Abdominal pain, pain during sexual intercourse and ectopic pregnancy. Miscarriages, sickly or premature babies, premature detachment of the placenta (abrupto placentae). Babies born to infected women suffer eye, ear, genital and lung infections; estimated that 25 percent of babies passing down infected birth canal will get chlamydia pneumonia and 50 percent chlamydia conjunctivitis a week after birth. In severe cases blindness occurs.
Gonorrhoea Second only to chlamydia in the number of reported cases. Generally found in the mucus areas of the body; genital tract, penis, rectum, vagina and throat.	In men: creamy or green pus-like discharge from penis, burning sensation with urination, testicular pain. In women: bleeding between periods, yellow or bloody discharge from vagina, heavy periods, bleeding associated with sexual intercourse, lower abdominal pain. Eighty percent of women and 10–15 percent of men show no symptoms at all.	Course of antibiotics. Scar tissue in the fallopian tubes, ectopic pregnancy, miscarriages. Inflammation of the testes leading to sterility.
Syphilis Caused by a bacterium treponema pallidum.	Early symptoms of syphilis are often very mild, and treatment is often not sought when first infected. Syphilis increases the risk of transmitting and receiving HIV. It can be passed on to others for up to 18 months. Secondary symptoms include rash, red lesions over the body, fever, swollen glands, lumps or warts.	Course of antibiotics. Over time, the bacteria move throughout the body, causing damage to many organs if untreated. Causes blindness, mental disorders and neurological disorders. 25 percent of pregnant women with active syphilis will have stillbirths or neonatal deaths, 40–70 percent will have syphilis-infected babies.
Thrush Caused by the yeast candida albicans, 50 percent of healthy sexually active women and 33 percent of pregnant women test positive for infection. Overgrowth of naturally occurring yeast can be due to fatigue, stress, 'the pill', poor diet or hygiene, tight clothing.	Vary from mild to severe. In women itching, burning, thick white cheesy discharge from the vagina, pain during sex and discomfort on passing urine, odour, vulva redness and swelling. In men: burning sensation during intercourse, transient rash, blisters, itching pain.	Cream, pessary or a single dose tablet. Dietary changes are essential for treating candida. Avoid alcohol, caffeine, dairy products, junk foods, sugar and white flour. Recurrence of infection.

In a recent survey of both partners in a London clinic, 69 percent were found to have at least one of the STDs listed on the left. In another survey 81 percent of the women were found to have one or more.

tubes with bacteria and white blood cells. Eventually, the body wins and the bacteria are controlled and destroyed. However, during the healing process, the delicate inner lining of the tubes is permanently scarred. The end of the tube by the ovaries may become partially or completely blocked, and scar tissue often forms on the outside of the tubes and ovaries. All these factors can impact on ovarian or tubal function and the chances of conception in the future.

Diagnosis

Tubal problems are investigated using a hysterosalpingogram (HSG) test in which a contrast fluid is injected through the cervix into the uterine cavity and down the fallopian tubes. The passage of this fluid is recorded on an x-ray. The fluid should pass rapidly out of both tubes if the tubes are functioning normally. Also a laparoscopy may be performed. A laparoscopy is when a fine telescope is inserted into the abdomen under general anaesthetic and enables the physician to view the external health of the tubes and look for any abnormalities like distortion caused by adhesions or infection. These tests are discussed in more detail in chapter 2.

Conventional treatment

If the fallopian tubes are damaged in any way, the chances of getting pregnant naturally decrease and the risk of ectopic pregnancy increases. Tubal surgery may be performed depending on the nature of the tubal damage. The chance of success will depend on the site of the blockage, presence of adhesions, age of the patient and whether tubal surgery has been attempted before.

It is important that each couple is fully investigated prior to surgery. The female partner needs her hormone profile checked, ovulation confirmed and a post coital test to exclude any sperm/mucus hostility. The male partner should have a semen analysis performed. If any additional problems are identified the option of IVF (in vitro fertilisation) should be considered. IVF bypasses the area of damage and avoids the risk of ectopic pregnancy. The egg is removed from the ovaries, fertilisation occurs in a test tube and the embryo is placed directly into the uterus for implantation.

Complementary treatment

If the tubes are completely blocked you will need the assistance of surgery or IVF to have a baby. However, if there is minimal damage to a fallopian tube, or one or both tubes are still functioning, you can take measures to ensure that further infections do not occur. After a course of antibiotics to 'kill' the infection, eating a healthy balanced diet will build up the reserves of essential nutrients.

The risk of ectopic pregnancy remains (see page 59). If a natural pregnancy occurs, a scan at six weeks will confirm the site of implantation in most cases.

OVULATION PROBLEMS

Healthy women will ovulate once a month about twelve times a year. For a woman who has irregular or absent periods, this may indicate that ovulation may be irregular or absent too, and, therefore, she will find it difficult to conceive that month.

The most common reasons ovulation does not take place are:
• PCOS or polycystic ovary syndrome
• Diminished ovarian reserve
• Premature ovarian failure
• Hormonal imbalances

PCOS (Polycystic Ovarian Syndrome)

This is a disorder of ovulation and is responsible for around 75 percent of cases of women with ovulation problems. These women usually have plenty of egg-containing follicles in their ovaries, but for hormonal reasons are unable to release eggs on a regular basis. This leads to the formation of empty egg follicles on the ovary, called cysts. Usually women with PCOS have 10 or more empty follicles, hence the name polycystic ovaries.

Cause

PCOS is a complex disorder in which a number of factors produce the polycystic ovary and trigger the symptoms. Factors thought to contribute are:

Insulin – a hormone that controls blood sugar level. Women with PCOS have high levels of insulin, which also stimulates an increase in the ovarian manufacture of testosterone, subsequently interfering with the normal development of follicles.

LH (Luteinising hormone) 40 percent of women with PCOS have raised LH levels, which could interfere with the development of the egg within the ovarian follicles. Too much LH might account for the increased production of testosterone.

Genetic PCOS tends to run in families. It is thought that one or more genes may make your ovaries more sensitive to insulin or LH.

Overweight excess fat can cause levels of insulin to rise. It is not known whether the weight contributes to PCOS or is a symptom of PCOS.

Symptoms

Women with PCOS may show the 'classic signs' – irregular or absent periods, acne, overgrowth of facial hair, hair loss from the scalp, being overweight and infertility. Symptoms may appear as early as late teens or early 20s and can vary from mild to severe. Not all symptoms occur in all women with PCOS, making it hard to diagnose. Other symptoms include depression, pelvic pain, breast pain, dizziness, bloating and mood swings, and recurrent miscarriage. On examination, the ovaries will be enlarged as they contain twice as many follicles as normal.

Diagnosis

Diagnosing PCOS can be difficult as women have differing symptoms with varying degrees of severity and may be unsure why they feel unwell or have irregular periods. It may help to keep a symptom diary for a couple of months prior to seeing the doctor to give a more accurate overview of your monthly cycle.

Monitoring BBT (the Basal Body Temperature) every month will highlight if you are ovulating regularly. A rise in temperature (usually between day 14 to 16 of a 28-day cycle) of about 0.5°C indicates that a surge in LH (luteinizing hormone) has occurred and ovulation is taking place. A sample BBT chart can be found on page 74 for you to start using.

If periods are irregular, your doctor may request an ultrasound scan of your ovaries and a blood test to measure hormone levels. Signs that PCOS may be present include elevated testosterone levels, elevated LH levels accompanied by normal or low FSH (follicle stimulating hormone) levels, elevated insulin levels and abnormal lipid (blood fats) profile.

Conventional treatment

One of the difficulties for PCOS sufferers is knowing when, and if, ovulation has taken place so they can actively have sex at the right time. Ovulation predictor kits do not work for women with PCOS as they may show a false positive due to the high levels of LH present. If pregnancy has not occurred naturally, fortunately most women with PCOS are able to get pregnant by stimulating ovulation with drugs like clomiphene citrate (clomid). It works by encouraging the body to produce its own supply of FSH. Usually tablets taken for 5 days after the start of the period is sufficient to stimulate the body. This is successful for 75 percent of women

SARAH'S STORY

I first raised questions as to my fertility in my late teens/early 20s. I never had established regular periods and although I gave it very little thought, in the back of my mind I always suspected that getting pregnant would not be easy for me.

It wasn't until planning my wedding in 1999 that I started to investigate the cause of my irregular cycle further. At this time a lot of my husband's friends were having children and we started to talk more about having a family in the future. As I had taken the pill for a while (this masked the problem and gave me a regular 28-day cycle), I decided to stop to see whether my cycle had become regulated. I found that this was not the case (I was going up to four months without a period) and also found that my skin broke out in spots and I was putting on weight.

Around this time, I came across a magazine article on PCOS. It all clicked into place, I had a lot of the symptoms the article mentioned. I went along to my GP but as we were not trying for a baby at the time he was not really interested. He dismissed the idea of PCOS, in his words, 'You don't look like a PCOS suffer. You don't look fat or hairy enough.'

Eventually, I went along to another GP. This time I was taken more seriously and referred for an ultrasound scan and blood tests. The scan showed that my ovaries were covered in follicular cysts. The explanation given was that the root cause of PCOS is insulin resistance. High levels of insulin stimulate the ovaries to produce excess testosterone. This testosterone can prevent the ovaries from releasing an egg each month, it is this that causes the follicular cysts. The blood tests proved that I had excess testosterone and it was this that was also causing some of my other symptoms – weight gain, acne, tiredness and mood swings. The doctor prescribed the contraceptive pill. This worked in masking the symptoms but did nothing to improve my fertility.

After we had been married for about a year, we decided I should stop taking the pill. For a while we were happy to leave it to fate but after a year of trying with no success, we started to wonder whether we would ever have children. We decided to try more actively but the problem with PCOS is that ovulation is infrequent so there is no way of identifying fertile days. This meant having sex every other day which was fun for a while but with stressful jobs and other things going on in life, the novelty soon wore off.

I visited my GP again but she explained that it takes many couples over a year to conceive with their first child so they would not start to investigate until we had been trying for 18 months. By this time the effect of sex every other day was starting to take its toll. Although we tried to keep a sense of humour, it was disheartening to find that if we took a couple of nights off – sometimes my period would arrive 14 days later – we had missed the chance! I started to investigate more about PCOS and began to understand the link between insulin resistance, hormonal imbalances and diet.

After a few months of making some dietary changes, I started to notice an improvement in my cycle. Finally, just as an appointment came through to see a specialist, I found out I was pregnant. My first son, Sam, was born in 2002.

Self-help for PCOS

Losing weight if you are overweight can help reduce insulin levels. By reducing insulin levels, testosterone levels will also reduce. This increases the likelihood of ovulation occurring and reduces other symptoms like hair growth and acne.

Diet has played a large part in helping PCOS sufferers overcome their problems and become pregnant. The diet should comprise of:

Protein such as lean meat, fish (an excellent source of omega 3 fatty acids which are important for those with PCOS), poultry, nuts, seeds, beans, lentils, dairy products, eggs and cheese.

Carbohydrates should make up about 50% of your daily calories in the complex form. Foods like fruit and vegetables, whole grains, such as brown rice, cereal, and wholemeal bread. Refined carbohydrates, white flour, sugar and caffeine should be eliminated from the diet.

Fibre helps maintain blood sugar balance. Without enough fibre, symptoms like weight gain, raised cholesterol, excess testosterone and oestrogen are likely to get worse. Sources of fibre include wholegrain seeds, nuts, fruits and vegetables or fibre supplements.

Essential fatty Acids (EFAs) include Omega-3 and Omega-6 fatty acids, and helps to regulate hormone function. Include olive oil, avocado, flaxseed oil, and oily fish like mackerel, salmon and sardines, as well as nuts, cashews, sunflower and pumpkin seeds. Avoid the saturated animal fats or transfatty acids often found in margarine, takeaways, peanut butter, and mayonnaise.

Lots of water – the body functions at its optimum on about eight glasses of water a day.

Further information on the PCOS diet can be found on page 89.

Exercise improves how the body metabolises insulin. In particular resistance training (weights, swimming, yoga) is said to build muscle, which increases the body's insulin sensitivity. On the other hand, cardiovascular exercise raises insulin levels and should be kept to a minimum.

Acupuncture and reflexology have shown promising results in women with mild polycystic ovarian syndrome in regulating their periods and inducing ovulation. More information on the benefits of acupuncture and reflexology in treating PCOS can be found in step 3.

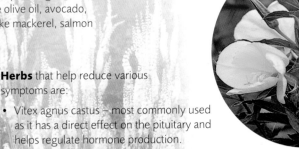

Herbs that help reduce various symptoms are:

- Vitex agnus castus – most commonly used as it has a direct effect on the pituitary and helps regulate hormone production.

- Dong Quai –helps with irregular menstruation, PMS, period pain and menopausal symptoms.

- Black Cohosh – helps with amenorrhoea, irregular menstruation and PMS. Can also help to lower blood pressure.

- Evening primrose – helps with irregular periods. It is rich in essential fatty acids, which the body requires to regulate hormones.

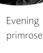

Evening primrose

A woman is born with her entire egg supply and, as time passes, these eggs become less viable. Approximately one third of women who wait until their mid- to late-30s to conceive will experience fertility problems.

with PCOS. If a response does not occur, FSH may be given by injection at specialised clinics. The response to clomid or FSH is much better in women of normal weight compared with those who are overweight.

Complementary treatment
There has been a lot of research and books published on holistic ways of approaching PCOS and increasing fertility (see box, opposite).

Diminished ovarian reserve

This is a condition in which women experience normal ovulation and menstrual cycles, but their ovaries do not respond normally to the hormones that allow conception to take place. Some view it as a precursor to ovarian failure or menopause. The age of the woman is a significant fertility factor. The chance of pregnancy for a woman aged 40 years and over is only five percent per menstrual cycle. It is known that the quality and quantity of eggs diminishes with age.

Other difficulties for the older woman include increased risk of miscarriage and genetic abnormalities in the unborn baby. More and more women are delaying trying for a baby and may not be aware of the consequences.

Diagnosis
A blood test measures the FSH (follicle stimulating hormone) and oestrogen levels on the third day of the menstrual cycle. FSH, together with LH (luteinizing hormone), controls oestrogen production from the ovaries. A result

that shows an elevated FSH means the pituitary gland is sending a frenzy of signals to the ovaries to get them to function, but that the ovaries in turn are not responding well. A normal FSH but high oestrogen level on day 3 is also not promising. This paradoxical finding suggests that the oestrogen level is too high early in the cycle, which in turn suppresses the FSH. It is generally agreed among medical professionals that FSH levels of higher than 12 mIU/mL on day 3 or oestrogen levels of higher than 50 to 60 pg/ml indicate at least some evidence of diminished ovarian reserve.

Conventional treatment
Hormonal therapies such as clomiphene citrate combined with IUI (intrauterine insemination) have been successful in patients under 40 with diminished ovarian reserve. In vitro fertilisation remains the most effective therapy for women using their own eggs but the live birth rate drops off considerably in women in their 40's. Unfortunately, there is no treatment that can restore eggs or improve their quality. Thus, it is critical to make sure a couple chooses the right clinic to assist them in conceiving from the beginning. With limited supplies, you will want to achieve the best chance of success first or second time round. How to choose the right clinic is discussed in detail in step 3.

Useful terms

Oligoovulation – irregular ovulation

Anovulation – lack of ovulation

Amenorrhoea – no menstrual cycle

Menorrhagia – excessive menstrual bleed

Dysmenorrhoea – painful menstruation

MARINA'S STORY

High FSH levels! ... Playing the waiting game
I decided that I would like another baby. Knowing that my only option is IVF as both of my fallopian tubes have been removed, I started the process with my clinic and had the initial hormone test performed between day 1–3 of my cycle. Little did I know of what lay ahead!

Since I conceived Bruno at 37 years old, my body has changed – I am two years older and it appears that my egg quality and quantity are showing signs of diminishing. This is maybe sooner than most women as, after all, I have stimulated my ovaries over the last five years through IVF, which has resulted in over 52 eggs being released in addition to the normal egg every month. Nevertheless, I am playing the waiting game. Waiting for the ideal month to arrive so that I can progress with IVF treatment. Most clinics require the hormones to be at an ideal level (FSH of 10 or below) as much evidence suggests that anything above this figure results in a poor ovarian response, poor egg quality and increased chance of miscarriage. So here I am, after three months of testing on day one of my monthly cycle praying my hormone levels reduce so I can try for another baby.

Now I am putting into practice everything I know and trying to level out my hormones. This includes following a wholefood diet similar to PCOS which focuses on lowering oestrogen levels, taking vitamin and herb supplements like agnus castus, vitamin B and zinc supplements and of course detoxing, which means my liver will be able to effectively remove 'old' hormones in my body. One theory is that is the body does not eliminate the monthly hormones that can accumulate month on month. Also, three months ago I had a Body Mass Index (BMI) of 18.4 which is deemed underweight for my height and evidence shows that being under- or over-weight can affect your hormone levels, so I have put on 3 kg (6.6 lbs), and now I have a BMI of 19.3 which is more in line with the normal range for my height. I've also had a reflexology session in which I developed a really bad headache. My reflexologist suggested that maybe my body was alleviating a blockage. Within an hour I felt fine, headache gone and I was overcome with a sense of calm. Now I am waiting for next week, day one of the fourth month of testing. Wish me luck!

Here is a summary of what my hormones are up to:

Year	Jan 03	May 05	July 05	Aug 05	Sep 05	Ideal conditions
Day of cycle	4	2	3	1	1	3
FSH level	9.5	12.7	9.9	10.1	8.6	below 10 iu/L
Oestradiol level	162	169	222	196	134	25.75pg/ml

▲ Conceived Bruno with these levels

(One week later ... All the hard work has paid off! My blood test results show both hormones at an all time low – even lower than two years ago when I conceived Bruno. I definitely think that putting on weight, re-balancing my hormones with supplements, and reflexology did the trick. I'm excited about the idea of trying for another baby now!)

POF (Premature Ovarian Failure)

Also known as premature menopause, this is a condition that results in what is essentially menopause in women younger than 35 years. It affects approximately one to four percent of females. Usually, women are born with enough eggs in their ovaries to ovulate one egg a month from puberty until about age 50 but for a woman diagnosed with POF, something has happened to her egg supply at a young age. It could be a lack of eggs, a problem with the eggs or follicles or the removal of her ovaries. Unlike menopause this is not a natural occurrence. Although the exact cause of POF is unknown, multiple factors are deemed to be involved including genetics, removal of ovaries, viral infection and even autoimmune disorders (when the body's own immune system attacks the ovary).

Finding out you have premature ovarian failure is devastating. Usually before you have even had a chance to consider having children, the choice has been taken away from you.

Symptoms

Women stop having their periods but experience hot flushes or night sweats, sleeping problems, mood swings, vaginal dryness, energy loss, low sex drive and painful sex. Other side effects are osteoporosis, diabetes and thyroid problems.

Diagnosis

A blood test to measure the level of FSH hormone will be taken for two to three consecutive months. Normal FSH levels are 10–15 mIU/ml and under; women with POF often have levels above 40 mIU/ml.

Treatment

HRT (hormone replacement therapy) is given but at this stage there is no treatment to restore fertility. If you wish to have a child, options include egg donation, adoption and surrogacy.

Hormonal imbalances

These can lead to a failure to ovulate, as a woman may be producing too much or too little of certain hormones. The primary glands (hypothalamus, pituitary and thyroid) are responsible for producing reproductive hormones. The hypothalamus, pituitary gland and ovaries send signals back and forth during the reproductive cycle that cause changes in hormone production. The hypothalamus can be affected by stress and some medications. An underactive thyroid causes hypothyroidism, which is characterised by excessive levels of prolactin, which interfere with ovulation.

Diagnosis

Hormonal imbalances are not hard to detect and treatment is relatively straightforward and effective in correcting the imbalance. A simple blood test will measure the prolactin levels and thyroid function.

Conventional treatment

Drugs like Parlodel can reduce raised prolactin levels. Synthetic thyroxine taken daily will help an underactive thyroid.

Endometriosis

This is very common and affects approximately two million girls and women in the UK.

The endometrium is the tissue that lines the uterus and increases in thickness during the menstrual cycle ready for the fertilised egg to implant. If pregnancy does not occur, the lining is shed as a 'period'. Endometriosis is a condition in which the endometrial cells start to grow outside their normal location inside the uterus.

These misplaced endometrial cells respond to the menstrual cycle in the same way as those lining the uterus. The tissue grows and sheds blood at the time of menstruation. However, instead of flowing out of the body through the vagina, the blood shed by the misplaced cells has no way of leaving the body. The resulting internal bleeding can lead to chronic inflammation and the formation of adhesions and

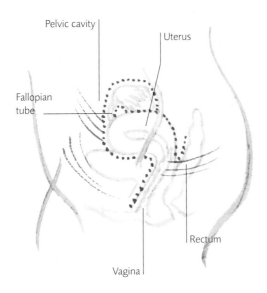

Pelvic cavity

Uterus

Fallopian tube

Rectum

Vagina

AREAS COMMONLY INFECTED BY ENDOMETRIOSIS
These include the ovaries, fallopian tubes, the ligaments that support the uterus, the area between the vagina and rectum, the outer surface of the uterus and the lining of the pelvic cavity.

scar tissue. Endometrial lesions can also be found in the bladder, bowel, vagina, cervix and vulva. More rarely the lung and other body tissues can be affected. Endometriosis affects eight to 10 percent of women of reproductive age.

Causes
The exact cause of endometriosis is unknown. More than one factor is likely to be involved. Theories under current consideration include:

Retrograde menstruation The oldest theory is that blood and endometrial cells back up from the uterus through the fallopian tubes, and enter the pelvic and abdominal cavities instead of flowing through the cervix and vagina. This migration process occurs in all women, though an immune or hormonal problem may allow the tissue to grow in the women who go on to develop endometriosis. The theory does not explain why women who undergo tubal ligation or hysterectomy can still experience symptoms of endometriosis.

Immunological changes These have been observed in women with endometriosis and have led to the theory that an abnormality in the immune system allows the endometrial cells that are shed normally to attach elsewhere and to grow. It is uncertain whether the

immunological changes are responsible for the endometriosis or the result of the inflammation caused by the disease.

Genetic Endometriosis tends to run in families, though the mode of inheritance remains unknown. Women with an affected mother or sister are more likely to have severe endometriosis than those without affected relatives.

Congenital factors Endometriosis may have existed from birth. During fetal development, uterine tissue may remain in the pelvis and grow as a result of hormonal influence.

Environmental causes There may also be a link between exposure to chemicals or allergens and endometriosis. Research on rhesus monkeys shows a link between exposure to dioxin and endometriosis. The greater the exposure to dioxin, the more severe the endometriosis. Dioxin is a by-product of pesticide and bleached pulp and paper products manufacturing. The chemical can also be produced through the burning of hazardous waste.

Symptoms
Some women with endometriosis have no symptoms; others can experience debilitating pain. Pelvic pain that is typical of endometriosis includes menstrual cramps, pain starting before periods, ovulation pain, low back pain that worsens during menstruation, painful and heavy periods with/without clots, premenstrual spotting and loss of dark or old blood before or at the end of a period. Pain in the pelvis may occur during or after sexual intercourse. Depending on where the implants are located, a woman may have painful bowel movements, bleeding from the bowel, pain when passing urine and

symptoms of irritable bowel (diarrhoea, constipation) in her rectum, painful urination and bowel movements during periods.

Diagnosis

A laparoscopy is the most conclusive diagnostic tool for evaluating if a woman has endometriosis. This is an operation in which a telescope (a laparoscope) is inserted into the pelvis via a small cut near the navel. This allows the surgeon to see the pelvic organs and any endometrial implants and cysts. Scans, blood tests and internal examinations are not a conclusive way to diagnose endometriosis. In 1994 the Endometriosis Society carried out a survey among its members, which revealed that the average time between first reporting symptoms and receiving a diagnosis was seven years.

Conventional treatment

The treatments available are aimed at removing the endometrial tissue, restoring fertility and preventing the reoccurrence of the condition; unfortunately there is no cure for endometriosis. Hormonal treatment is designed to stop ovulation and allow the endometrial deposits to die off. The preferred option for women trying to conceive is to undergo laparoscopy during which the endometrial tissue is removed. In severe cases, a hysterectomy may be advised to alleviate the debilitating symptoms. You should discuss this in great detail with your gynaecologist and explore any other options, as once your uterus is removed your chances for having a baby are zero!

Complementary treatment

As high levels of oestrogen may contribute to endometriosis, a diet that limits the amount of oestrogen you ingest is advisable. This diet is the same as that recommended for PCOS and other hormonal imbalances (see page 91).

UTERINE PROBLEMS

There are a number of problems affecting the uterus and/or its lining that can cause or contribute to infertility or recurrent miscarriage.

Uterine fibroids

These are benign growths (non-cancerous), which grow from cells forming the muscle of the uterus. About 25 percent of women of childbearing age have uterine fibroids and they are most common in 30- to 50-year-old women. With the trend towards delayed childbearing, more and more women are encountering the problems of fibroids during their reproductive years. These tumours grow in various locations on and within the uterine wall or in the uterine cavity. No one is certain what causes uterine fibroids but changing oestrogen levels seem to play a part in their growth. When oestrogen levels are high – as a result of pregnancy or the contraceptive pill, for example – the rate of fibroid growth increases. As a woman approaches the menopause and her oestrogen levels get lower, uterine fibroids are likely to shrink or almost disappear. Besides being a woman of reproductive age, no other risk factors for fibroids have been found.

Symptoms

A women can live with fibroids for years without having any symptoms or being aware of their presence. Others may become aware of them as a result of recurrent miscarriages; they are able to conceive easily but miscarry early on, as the fertilised egg is unable to grow with a fibroid present. Symptoms include heavy bleeding, prolonged periods, bleeding between periods, pain, increased need for urination, pressure on the rectum with constipation and lower back and abdominal pain.

Diagnosis

Most uterine fibroids are found during a routine internal examination when the doctor notices a lumpy or irregular uterus. If symptoms are painful or recurring, the GP may arrange for an ultrasound to distinguish fibroids from cysts, tumours and other pelvic masses.

Conventional treatment

Most fibroids do not need to be treated as they may disappear on their own. The doctor will make a decision to surgically remove them based on the rate of growth, amount of pain or blood loss, age and desire to have children. Myomectomy is the term used to refer to the surgical removal of fibroids. Depending upon the location of the fibroid, myomectomy can be accomplished by either an abdominal or vaginal approach.

If the cause of infertility is diagnosed as fibroids, evidence suggests that fertility may be restored after surgery. A study of 94 infertile women with uterine fibroids who had at least one tumour larger than 3 cm (1¼ in) and no other apparent cause for infertility, showed that following surgical removal of fibroids, 59.5 percent of these women conceived, most within a short time. The miscarriage rate in the presence of fibroids is about 40 percent. Following surgery, 80 percent of patients with a history of repeated miscarriages will have a successful pregnancy.

Even after a myomectomy, there is a 25 percent chance that new fibroids will grow within 10 years of surgery. The only procedure that almost guarantees fibroids will not recur is a hysterectomy. A hysterectomy used to be the standard treatment for uterine fibroids, the procedure is now only recommended for women who are nearly at the menopause, are not concerned with having children or have very severe symptoms.

Complementary treatment

It is thought that fibroids respond to the same treatment as endometriosis and PCOS, as each condition is a result of too much oestrogen in the body. A woman who changes from a high-fat high-protein diet to a low-fat high-fibre, mostly vegetarian, diet will experience decreased bleeding and even a decrease in the size of her fibroid. A detailed overview of the diet can be found in step 3. In summary, the highlights of what is recommended are:

- Cut out red meat and animal products as they stimulate oestrogen overproduction
- Take Lactobacillus acidophilus supplements to prevent reabsorption of hormones.
- Increase fibre intake as it reduces oestrogen levels by preventing reabsorption. Women who eat a vegetarian diet excrete three times more 'old', detoxified oestrogens than women

who eat meat. The meat eaters also reabsorb more oestrogen.

- Reduce or eliminate sugar as it increases fat, which subsequently increases oestrogen production.
- Eliminate alcohol as it compromises the efficiency of the liver in metabolising hormones.
- Agnus castus, is one of the most important herbs for female hormone problems. It restores hormonal balance.
- Milk thistle works on improving liver function.
- Dandelion also helps cleanse the liver and rid the body of old female hormones.

Uterine polyp

This is an overgrowth of tissue in the lining of the uterus. Small polyps generally do not interfere with reproductive abilities, however large polyps – or multiple polyps – can interfere with conception and may increase the risk of miscarriage.

Symptoms
Irregular bleeding, heavy bleeding between periods, spotting.

Diagnosis
Doctors may use an HSG (hysterosalpingogram) to take an x-ray of the uterus and fallopian tubes to see if there are any polyps. A hysteroscopy is another common diagnostic procedure that many doctors use, in which a small tube is inserted into the uterus through the vagina, allowing a visual examination of the area.

Treatment
Removing polyps is fairly simple. A hysteroscope is used to guide your doctor to the area and scrape the polyp from the uterus. Some women experience some spotting for a few days after the procedure and are able to return to normal activities within a few days. Fertility should return to normal after the polyps have been removed.

Intrauterine adhesions

Often referred to Asherman's syndrome, scar tissue can interfere with reproductive functions by preventing conception and increasing the risk of miscarriage. It is uncommon. The scar tissue may be a result of an infection acquired after having had a D&C (dilation and curettage) or a miscarriage or abortion. The treatment is similar to removal of polyps, in which a hysteroscope is used to cut through any adhesions.

Congenital malformations

Some women are born with malformed uteruses, which make conceiving and carrying a pregnancy to full term difficult.

A bicornate uterus is where the woman has a heart-shaped, instead of pear shaped, uterus, which means the fetus is unable to grow as the uterus does not expand.

A septate uterus has a wall inside the uterus that divides the cavity. Although many women with this condition do not have any trouble conceiving and carrying a pregnancy to term, one in four will experience repeat miscarriages. However, this condition can be successfully treated through a hysteroscopy or laparoscopy. About 80 percent of the women who have had their septum removed have been able to carry a pregnancy to term.

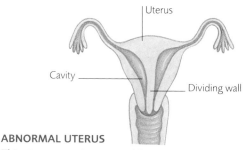

Uterus

Cavity

Dividing wall

ABNORMAL UTERUS
This uterus contains two cavities but it may be able to support a pregnancy should an egg implant.

MALE FACTORS

When a couple fails to conceive, the male is responsible almost as often as the female. Male infertility is said to be on the increase as sperm counts have reduced by 53 percent in the last 50 years. A study in 1992 found that men in Western countries today have less than half the sperm production their grandfathers had at the same age. The study concluded that there had been a 42 percent decrease in average sperm count, from 113 million per millilitre (ml) to 66 million per ml, since 1940. Furthermore, the average volume of semen diminished from 3.4 ml to 2.75 ml, a 20 percent loss since 1940.

In addition, when the European Society for Human Reproduction and Embryology evaluated couples undergoing fertility treatment in 24 countries, it became clear that treatment for male infertility had risen. ICSI (intracytoplasmic injection) treatment in which a single sperm is injected directly into an egg, accounted for 43 percent of IVF cycles in 1997 and 52 percent in 2002. It appears that the causes of infertility are shifting away from the previous dominant cause, female tubal disease towards male factor infertility. One theory suggests this may be due to the fact that in the last 15 years sex protection (with the increased awareness of AIDS) has reduced the incidence of STDs, and subsequently tubal disease, whereas there has been an increase in environmental toxins and a shift in diet and lifestyle, which have affected sperm production.

Sperm counts are not the only aspect to be affected; sperm quality and motility have also been compromised. A 20-year study published in 1995 in the *New England Journal of Medicine* reported a decline of 0.6 percent of motile sperm and a 0.5 percent decline in the proportion of healthy sperm per year. A European study reported a staggering decline in sperm counts of 3.1 percent each year between 1971 and 1990. The evidence is compelling.

What are the causes of male infertility?
Male infertility can be classified into two areas: problems associated with sperm production and problems with sperm delivery. Sperm production

Sperm has to travel about three to four inches to fertilise an egg; this is the human equivalent of about 26 miles – a marathon!

problems account for the majority of male infertility and are concerned with the amount of sperm produced, their shape and structure (morphology) and ability to swim (motility). If any of these aspects are below average, fertilisation becomes more difficult.

SPERM PRODUCTION PROBLEMS

A low sperm count is considered to be one less than 20 million sperm per ml of semen. Below five million, a man is definitely sterile. Motility describes the proportion of moving sperm. A normal sample will contain at least 50 percent rapidly moving sperm in straight lines with some erratic behaviour. If the sperm are twitching or not moving at all, it indicates a fertility problem.

So why are we seeing a decline in sperm counts? There are many factors that may contribute to a reduction in quantity and quality of sperm such as excessive heat resulting in varicocele, nutritional and environmental factors and stress.

Varicocele

Varicocele is a term used to describe a condition where there are enlarged varicose veins around the testicle and vas deferens that cause abnormalities in the temperature regulation of the testis. About 20 percent of fertile men have varicocele but twice as many infertile men have it. In 90 percent of cases it is on the left-hand side. It is the most common identifiable cause of infertility in men.

Causes
Enzymes that are responsible for both sperm and hormone (testosterone) production have an optimal temperature at which they operate most effectively. If this temperature is elevated by even one degree, sperm and testosterone production is adversely affected.

Men can help to improve their fertility by ensuring their testes do not overheat. Common causes of this are soaking in hot baths, working in a high environmental temperature, taking regular jacuzzis and saunas and wearing too-tight underwear. Men whose jobs involve long hours of sitting, e.g. long distance lorry-drivers and travelling salesmen, may have reduced fertility due to the increased heat to their genital areas. Men who are overweight or obese naturally increase the temperature around the genital area with the excess body fat around the lower abdomen.

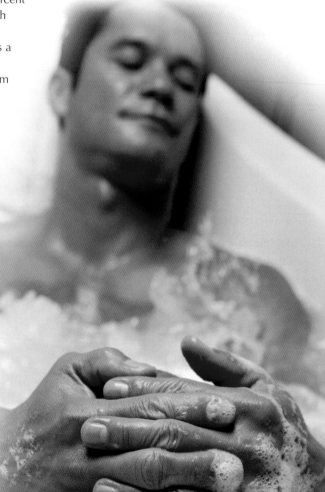

Treatment

Surgery is recommended for men with a varicocele if they suffer pain, damage or atrophy to the testicles or if treatment is required for sterility. The procedure involves tying off the distended veins under local or general anaesthetic. It takes about 90 days for a sufficient quantity of new sperm to be produced to permit fertilisation. Fifty percent of men who have a varicocelectomy to correct infertility father children within a year. Five to 20 percent who receive treatment for varicocele have a recurrence of the condition.

JOHN'S STORY

I had been told I had a very low sperm count and it was unlikely I would father a child. It was suggested that both my wife and I stopped smoking and drinking, though neither of us were heavy drinkers and I smoked only 10 cigarettes a day. We both agreed to a hair analysis and followed the Foresight dietary programme. It took about seven months for me to get a good zinc reading. Shortly after this my wife became pregnant and subsequently our little girl arrived, weighing 7 lb 7 oz.

Vital vitamins and minerals

Zinc plays an important role in the formation of new sperm and maintenance of sperm motility. A deficiency in zinc can result in a decreased sperm count or decreased motility causing infertility. For infertile men with low semen zinc levels, a preliminary trial found that zinc supplements (240 mg per day) increased sperm counts and possibly contributed to successful impregnation by three of the 11 men. In another controlled study, 100 men with low sperm motility received either 57mg of zinc twice daily or a placebo. After three months, there was significant improvement in those taking zinc: sperm quality, sperm count, sperm motility, and fertilising capacity of the sperm all increased.

Vitamin C protects sperm from oxidative damage and prevents sperm from sticking together – sperm agglutination. In one study, men who suffered agglutination took a supplement of 200 to 1,000 mg per day, which increased their fertility.

Arginine is needed to produce sperm. Research shows that several months of arginine supplementation increases sperm count, quality and fertility. However, if the sperm count is below 10 million per ml it seems to have no effect. Many doctors recommend supplementation of up to 4 grams per day for several months if sperm count levels are greater than 10 million per ml.

Vitamin B$_{12}$ is needed to maintain fertility. A study of infertile men showed that taking 1,500 mcg per day for 2 to 13 months increased the sperm counts in 60 percent of the men.

Vitamin E deficiency has shown to lead to infertility in animals. In a preliminary human trial, 100–200 IU of vitamin E given daily to both partners of infertile couples led to a significant increase in fertility. It is thought that vitamin E supplementation may enhance fertility by decreasing free radical damage to sperm cells.

Nutritional and environmental factors

Much research has been carried out in this field to ascertain how these factors can influence the health of sperm. It is known that healthy sperm need an abundance of nutrients and if these are not readily available the delicate process of spermatogenesis is affected.

Organic produce The case for eating organic food is mounting. In a study of Danish greenhouse workers, an unexpectedly high sperm count was found among organic farmers, who grew their products without the use of pesticides or chemical fertilisers. The sperm count was more than twice as high in these men as in a control group of blue-collar workers. Although these findings are not definitive, they suggest that consuming organically grown foods may enhance fertility.

Diagnosis

It is particularly difficult to assess if your body is deficient in essential vitamins and minerals or overloaded with harmful toxic chemicals. One method that is becoming increasingly popular is HMA (hair mineral analysis). A segment of hair can give an accurate history of what has been passed into the hair follicle in the previous six to eight weeks. This is useful as some minerals are only found in small amounts in the hair, reflecting the small amounts throughout the body, although they play a vital role in the body. Hair analysis is accurate down to 0.1 parts per million or less. Details of the benefits and results of a hair mineral analysis can be found in step 2.

Treatment

Vitamin supplementation is recommended if you are deficient in essential vitamins and minerals. Organisations like Foresight are able to create a vitamin supplementation programme specific to your requirements following hair analysis. A period of up to three months is recommended before re-analysing the hair to assess the improvements in your health.

Smoking and drinking

Smoking over 20 cigarettes a day has been shown to reduce both the sperm count and the sperm motility to quite a major degree. Excessive alcohol intake will lead to infertility mainly because a man loses both the inclination and the ability to rise to the occasion! Alcohol can also lower the production of sperm and of the male hormone testosterone. In a study of men with poor sperm quality, excessive alcohol consumption was associated with a decrease in the percentage of normal sperm.

The only treatment to advise is to give up smoking, drinking and drugs if you are serious about conceiving a baby. By doing so you will be maximising your chances of conception!

Illnesses and disorders

A variety of illnesses can affect the structure or quality of the sperm. Cystic fibrosis may cause absence of sperm, vas deferens, or seminal vesicles. Previous inflammation of the testes from mumps or high fever will affect sperm production and quality. Sexually transmitted diseases (STDs) cause obstruction, infection, and scarring. Antibiotics will clear the infection; however, if the infection has been left untreated for a period of time, it is likely to have caused some damage to the reproductive organs. If this is the case, a vasogram and/or testicular biopsy will assist in ascertaining the damage caused.

Presence of Antibodies

Sometimes, a semen sample when seen under a microscope, will show sperm clumping. If as a result of trauma or surgery, sperm has come into contact with the body's immune system antibodies may be produced. The clumping is a sign that sperm antibodies are present and will affect their ability to fertilise an egg.

Hormone Disorders

These are rare causes of male infertility, but it may sometimes be helpful to check the levels of FSH, LH, testosterone, prolactin and thyroid hormone.

Genetic disorders

Very small testicles may be the manifestation of this genetic abnormality in which the man has an extra x (female) chromosome know as Klinefelter's syndrome. Often a man with this condition produces no sperm at all and sperm donation is the fertility treatment offered.

Age

Until recently it has been widely thought that a man's reproductive capability was not affected by advancing age. There are many stories about men who have fathered children in their sixties and even as late as their nineties. Yet now figures show that men over 40 are making up nearly a quarter of fertility consultations. Until recently there has been a poor understanding of the effect of aging on male fertility. It is only now that the field of male infertility has become mainstream and full of new research, data and conclusions.

What happens? Whilst the effects of aging are not as dramatic as those seen in women, subtle changes in DNA quality could seriously affect a

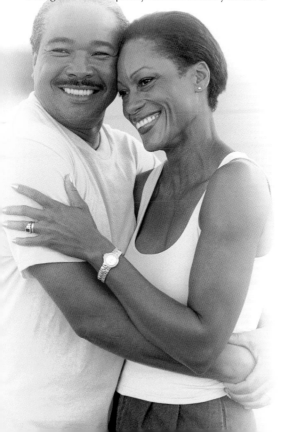

couple's ability to conceive, or could lead to miscarriage or even health problems in any children born.

A team of Canadian scientists found that damage to DNA in sperm increases with age. DNA damage was far higher in men over 45 than in younger men; men aged 45 had double the damage of those younger than 30. Another study analysed the sperm of 2,134 men and found a wide variation in quality that was linked with age.

Age has an effect on a man's ability to conceive. Increasingly, couples are leaving parenthood until later in life without realising the potential consequences and the price to be paid.

SPERM DELIVERY PROBLEMS

A number of conditions, such as blockages and obstructions, illness and Klinefelter's syndrome can also prevent the sperm reaching an egg.

Blockages and obstructions

The second major cause of infertility in men is blockages and obstructions of the male reproductive tract. It is important to ascertain which category a man falls into: is he making sperm, but a blockage or obstruction is preventing the sperm fertilising an egg or is he not producing sperm at all?

Cause

Blockage can be caused by a urinary tract infection or by a sexually transmitted disease such as chlamydia and gonorrhoea. Bacteria can infect the epididymis, which is essentially a swimming school for sperm before they are able to swim to fertilise an egg. Epididymitis can cause scarring and blockage, inhibiting the sperm from leaving the duct to fertilise an egg.

Diagnosis

A vasogram is an x-ray of the vas deferens, the tube connecting the testis with the seminal vesicles. Under general anaesthetic, a dye is injected into the vas deferens. If a blockage exists, the exact location will become apparent on an x-ray. A testicular biopsy may also be performed. A sample of tissue from the testicle is taken and examined for any abnormalities in sperm production or maturation. If sperm development appears normal yet semen analysis shows reduced or absent sperm, a blockage of the tube will be suspected.

Treatment

When a blockage has been identified, surgery may be required to repair or unblock the ducts so that sperm can be transported through the reproductive tract. If surgery cannot correct the blockage, sperm may be collected directly from the testis and be used for assisted reproduction.

MALE TREATMENTS

In summary, male infertility can be treated with techniques that circumvent the problem. Methods to assist conception include in vitro fertilisation where despite low number of normal motile sperm, fertilisation can occur as the sperm is placed in the immediate vicinity of the egg. Males with low sperm count and poor motility can have sperm retrieved surgically from the testes or epididymis. A revolutionary technique called ICSI (intracytoplasmic injection), where a single sperm is injected directly into the egg, has shown to have a 60–70 percent fertilisation success rate. The development of ICSI means that there are now very few men for whom there is no possibility of fathering their own children.

Very little progress has been made in finding the ultimate cause of reduced sperm counts and sperm motility. Drug treatments have done little to increase sperm concentration or sperm counts. In the last decade, a correlation between age and male infertility has been confirmed. In addition, the evidence to suggest that a change in your nutrition and lifestyle is an effective treatment for both male and female infertility is growing. Many eminent nutritionists advocate a healthy diet, free of alcohol, smoking and drugs to maximise the chances of conception.

Tubes may be blocked or retrograde ejaculation may occur

A man may suffer from erectile problems

Varicose veins in the scrotum may lower sperm count

Sperm may be malformed or be of low motility

The testicles may not produce sperm

Useful terms

Aspermia – The patient produces no sperm

Azoospermia – The patient produces semen containing no sperm

Oligospermia – Sperm concentration is low, less that 20 million per ml

Asthenospermia – Less than 50 percent of the sperm are active

Teratospermia – More than 70 percent of the sperm are abnormally shaped

Oligoasthenoteratozoospermia (OATS) – Less than 20 million sperm per ml with 50% being motile and more than 70 percent abnormally shaped

Necrospermia – All sperm are dead

Pyospermia or leucospermia – Presence of a large number of white blood cells in semen, often associated with infection

COUPLE FACTORS

Sometimes, it can't be ascertained whether it's the male or female who has a problem.

Unexplained infertility

This is the term used to classify couples in which standard infertility testing has not found a cause for the failure to conceive. Twenty percent of couples have unexplained infertility.

Why is this so high? It is important to realise that the medical profession has made huge inroads into understanding infertility in the last 30 years and has developed many ART (assisted reproductive technologies) to provide couples with children they otherwise would not have. However, there are still a lot of aspects that cannot be explained and require further research. The standard fertility tests look for obvious reasons for infertility like abnormal sperm counts, blocked tubes and ovulation irregularity. As I pointed out earlier, there are literally hundreds of molecular and biochemical processes that come into play for conception to take place. Fertility testing does not assess all these factors and therefore if standard testing has not shown an obvious cause, a couple is usually diagnosed with unexplained infertility.

Causes

Stress Typically, a couple have completed many fertility tests over a period of six months and have become frustrated about why they have not yet conceived. This additional stress can have a natural contraceptive effect on the mind-body connection. Add this to other factors such as bad nutrition, excess alcohol, smoking, low levels of the required vitamins and minerals and having sex at the wrong time, it is no wonder the body is not responding. These may sound obvious reasons but it is amazing how many couples that are actively trying for a baby fall into one of these categories.

Duration Research has shown that the longer the infertility, the less likely the couple is to conceive on their own; after 5 years of unexplained infertility, a couple has less than a 10 percent chance for success. Another study showed that for couples with unexplained infertility of over three years' duration, the cumulative conception rate after 24 months of attempting conception without any treatment was 28 percent. This number reduces by 10 percent for each year that the female is over 31. Other factors could also be contributing to the success rate such as egg quality and quantity as they diminish with advancing age.

Immunological causes Some research suggests that unexplained infertility could be due to immunological problems, which are hidden in the peritoneal fluid (the space between membranes in the abdominal cavity) away from routine sites of investigations. Further basic research is needed to define the specific role of peritoneal fluid cells, which may offer the possibility of more effective treatment of unexplained infertility.

Uterine blood flow Research shows that women with unexplained infertility have significantly reduced blood flow during all phases of the menstrual cycle compared to that of fertile women.

Conventional treatment

Your doctor may discuss a variety of treatments and options with you. These include ovarian stimulation methods, intrauterine insemination, IVF and ICSI. At this stage it is important to weigh up the pros and cons of each treatment, as there can be side effects of any treatment such as ovarian hyperstimulation, ectopic pregnancy and miscarriage (see page 56).

Many couples want a baby at any cost and will immediately try assisted reproductive technologies before complementary options. For couples under 35 with unexplained infertility, it may be wise to embark on a period of healthy living to see if you are able to conceive naturally before taking drugs and undergoing assisted reproductive methods. You may be surprised by the results!

Complementary treatment

Many couples diagnosed with unexplained infertility feel helpless. After all the fertility testing they are still unaware of what is wrong and what action they can take to increase their chances of getting pregnant. Organisations like Foresight have developed a highly successful whole food diet and vitamin supplementation programme to help couples achieve a successful pregnancy. A three-year study looked at couples that had previously suffered with primary and secondary infertility. All couples followed the whole food diet and vitamin supplementation programme and a staggering 86 percent of these couples became pregnant and gave birth to healthy babies. As these results are very encouraging it is worth looking at the study in greater detail. Three hundred and sixty-seven couples took part in the study; the average age for females was 34 years (22 to 45) and males 36 years (25 to 59).

What the study showed

Before embarking on the wholefood diet it was assessed that:

90 percent of the males and **60 percent** of the females regularly drank alcohol;

45 percent of the men and **57 percent** of the women smoked;

59 percent of the couples had a history of reproductive problems;

37 percent of the couples had suffered infertility for between 1 to 10 years;

38 percent of the women had histories of one to five miscarriages;

42 percent of the males had semen analysis due to infertility and most had a reduction in sperm quality;

3 percent of the women had given birth to a stillborn child.

Of the babies previously born alive, 40 were small for dates, 15 of low birth weight (less than 2.5 kg/5 lb 8 oz), 7 malformed and 3 died of SIDS (sudden infant death syndrome).

Common complaints of the prospective parents were fatigue, headaches or migraines, cold feet, back pain, abdominal bloating and constipation.

After completing the wholefood programme:

89 percent (327) of the women became pregnant, **100 percent** of whom delivered healthy babies. No miscarriages occurred and all babies were well developed at birth, average birth weight being 3.25 kg (6 lb 12 oz), and none were malformed or transferred to special baby-care units.

Among the 204 couple with infertility problems, **86 percent** had achieved healthy pregnancies.

These results clearly demonstrate that preconceptual care directly affects pregnancy outcome. The most sophisticated technologies achieve an average of only 25 percent success.

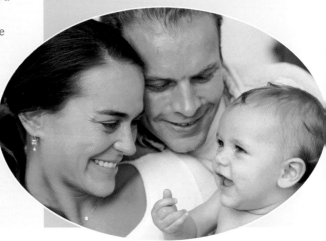

Age and fertility

Age and fertility is a topic that is difficult to tackle. Many of us do not want to acknowledge that we are growing old let alone discover the fact that our reproductive capabilities are waning. In my experience women fall into two categories: those that do not feel under pressure to reproduce until later in life versus women who are immensely conscious of their biological clock ticking. Unfortunately there are not many body signals to let you know that your reproductive potential is declining as you age. This is why many women are surprised to learn it may be too late or more difficult than anticipated. What women really need is a gauge on their bodies, like a petrol indicator, which shows when their tanks are half full so they can take action before it is too late!

Many women today are leaving child-bearing until later in life for a variety of reasons. The most common are a desire for a successful career and wanting to wait for a stable relationship or financial security. This is a good decision to make if you can be absolutely sure that you will be able to have children without any problems in the future.

In my case, my husband and I started trying when we were both 31 years old, which is still relatively young compared to most of our peers. We were unaware that we would meet with so many obstacles along the way and that it would take six years before our first child was born. When I became pregnant at the age of 37, other issues not considered risk factors at 31 entered

A woman's chronological age is not the same as her biological age. A woman may be 25 years old but have the reproductive capabilities of a 37-year-old or vice versa. A 44-year-old may be reproductively comparative to a 32-year-old. Two women with apparently normal cycles can have different levels of ovarian reserve.

the equation, such as diminishing egg quality and quantity, increased risk of chromosomal disorders and miscarriage.

If I were restricted to only one piece of advice in this book, it would be that a woman should find out her reproductive capability by assessing her ovarian reserve with a blood test in her 30s. FSH (follicle stimulating hormone) levels rise as a woman ages and women with abnormal FSH levels can have considerable difficulty conceiving with their own eggs. By having this test it may provide the evidence needed to either start trying for a baby straightaway or to delay having a baby until later.

Effects of age

All the eggs a woman ever produces are already present in her ovaries as a developing fetus as early as the 7th to 10th week of pregnancy. From then on there is a reduction with time. At eighteen weeks' gestation, there are 6 to 7 million; at birth 1 to 2 million and approximately

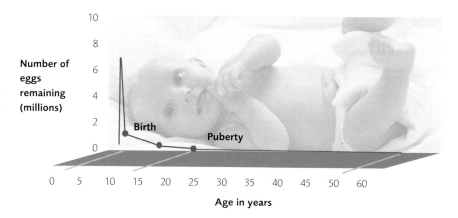

Number of eggs remaining (millions)

Birth

Puberty

0 5 10 15 20 25 30 35 40 45 50 60

Age in years

EGGS AND AGE
Over time, the number of eggs capable of being fertilised drops markedly.

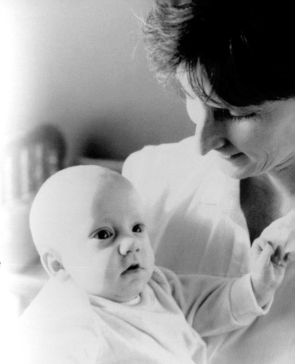

400,000 by the time she reaches puberty. The rate of loss continues until climacteric at about 50 years of age, when egg production ceases altogether.

This decline in egg quality and quantity with age affects a woman's ability to get pregnant, conceive a healthy baby free of chromosomal abnormalities and to carry a developing fetus to full term. Biological data suggests that at least three factors undergo change as a woman ages: at age 37, the uterus becomes increasingly unreceptive to maintaining pregnancy; a change in hormone patterns, marked by rising FSH levels, increases the incidence of menstrual dysfunction which leads to an inability to conceive; after age 45, embryo abnormalities (chromosomal trisomies) become dominant and compose half of all conceptions.

Other indications of reproductive aging are the shortening of the menstrual cycle. If the cycle was previously a typical 27 to 28 day cycle and has now shortened to 23 or 24 days, this could be a signal of diminishing ovarian reserve. It is thought that the eggs become a bit 'deaf' to hormonal signals from the pituitary gland. As a result, the pituitary starts sending signals earlier, which causes faster egg development and shorter cycles.

Chance of a normal pregnancy reduces The chart below highlights how the chance of getting pregnant each month begins to decrease in your 30s and markedly diminishes in your 40s.

Risk of miscarriage increases The risk of miscarriage at age 25 to 29 is 10 percent while the risk at age 40 to 44 is 34 percent.

In 2001 a study measured the ovarian reserve of 10,000 women of all ages. Ten percent of the

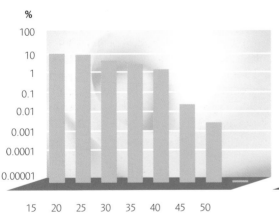

%

Age in years

EFFECT OF AGE ON PREGNANCY
Your ability to become pregnant remains fairly stable until the latter part of your 30s, when it decreases markedly.

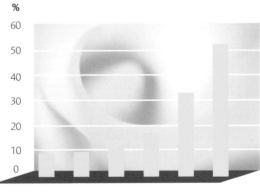

%

Age in years

AGE AND MISCARRIAGE
The older you are, the more likely you will be to experience an early end to pregnancy.

*It's not all doom and gloom.
Women who gave birth to one or
two children in their 30s and 40s
had a greater chance of living into
their 80s. The reasons were not
clear, although it may be that a
later pregnancy might mean later
menopause and a delayed onset
of age-related diseases such as
stroke and Alzheimer's.*

women had an abnormal ovarian reserve (raised
FSH levels). In this group there were only 28
pregnancies (2.7 percent of patients) with 20 of
them (71 percent) ending in miscarriage. The
eight patients with a child represent 0.7 percent
of the patients with abnormal ovarian reserve.
This confirms that regardless of age, an abnormal
ovarian reserve result indicates a dramatic
decrease in the ability to have a child.

Risk of chromosomal abnormality increases
The risk of chromosomal abnormality in a

% Abnormal

AGE AND FETAL ABNORMALITIES
*More babies with chromosomal
abnormalities are conceived by older
women.*

woman aged 20 years is 1 in 500 while the risk
in a woman aged 45 is 1 in 20.

Fetal chromosomal abnormalities account for
nearly 50 percent of early miscarriages. This may
be due to abnormalities in the egg, sperm or
both. The usual chromosomal pattern is 46
chromosomes, which are arranged in 23 pairs.
The most common chromosomal defects are
trisomy, where there are three chromosomes of
one type instead of the normal two. The risk of
having a Down's baby increases with age from
one in 400 at the age of 35 to one in 109 at age
40 and one in 32 after age 45. When a woman
is 35 or older, the doctor may recommend an
amniocentesis test be performed to measure the
baby's chromosomes and assess the risk of
disorders like Down's syndrome.

Other factors affected *Low birth weight*
It seems older mothers are more likely to have
a low-weight baby (less than 2.5 kg/5 lb 8 oz)
and much of this risk results from multiple
births. In 2000, 55 percent of low-birth-weight
babies with mothers over 45 were born in
multiple deliveries. Where just one baby was
born, women over 45 were substantially less
likely to have a low-birth-weight baby than
younger women.

Diabetes A recent study showed there is an
increased risk of first babies of older mothers
being at greater risk of diabetes. It was found that
the mother's age at delivery strongly related to
the risk of type 1 (insulin-dependent) diabetes.
The risk increased by 25 percent for each five-
year band, so a 45-year-old mother was more
than three times likely to have a child who
developed diabetes than a 20-year-old.

Stillbirth In 2000, a study into the effect of
conceiving later in life, using data from
Denmark, confirmed that age strongly increases
the chances of at least three undesirable
outcomes – miscarriage, ectopic pregnancy and
stillbirth. Nobody knows why, but there is a
greater incidence of stillbirth in women aged
over 35 right at the end of pregnancy: one in
440 babies in mature mothers as opposed to one
in 1000 for younger women.

CATHERINE'S STORY

I had just got married – aged 42 – and as I had no health problems that I knew of, I saw no reason why I could not have a baby! I followed the Foresight wholefood diet and had a tailored vitamin and mineral supplementation programme. The pregnancy took a little time to get under way but I stuck with the programme and remained optimistic. Just after my 44th birthday my little girl arrived weighing 7 lb 7 oz – very healthy, very lively and very beautiful!

Treatments

Unfortunately, there are no treatments available that can 'turn back the clock' on a woman's ovaries. Treatments for older women focus on stimulating the ovaries to produce an increased number of eggs in the hope that one will be healthy and viable for pregnancy. If the eggs are poor quality or there is an inadequate supply, egg donation may be discussed. The options include:

Controlled ovarian hyperstimulation This involves using drugs such as clomiphene citrate to encourage the ovaries to produce more eggs followed by IUI (intrauterine insemination) – a process where sperm are placed into the uterine cavity via a catheter.

IVF (In vitro fertilisation) This is the most effective treatment for women using their own eggs. The success rates diminish with age. Day 3 FSH (follicle stimulating hormone) levels have shown to be an accurate predictor of IVF success, independent of age. Every IVF clinic establishes a threshold FSH limit above which pregnancies are rarely conceived. This may vary from clinic to clinic, however most agree that levels above 15 predict that IVF will be of little value in helping achieve pregnancy.

Egg donation Women with high FSH levels are likely to be told that IVF will be unsuccessful. Fortunately women in this situation still have good options of becoming parents using an egg donor or adopting a child. Egg donation is the process whereby eggs from a young woman can be fertilised and placed into the uterus of an older woman. The egg is fertilised with her partner's sperm and inserted into the older woman's womb for implantation to take place.

Reports demonstrate that if you use younger eggs, the rate of achieving pregnancies in older women is very high. In fact, egg donation gives the highest rate of pregnancy that is achievable with any type of fertility. As compared to pregnancy rates of less than 10 percent per cycle for women over the age of forty, egg donation results in pregnancy rates of over 45 percent per cycle. In addition, the risks of miscarriage and Down's syndrome are dramatically reduced. This is excellent proof that fertility decreases with age due to the aging of the eggs and chromosomes.

Complementary treatments These can work in conjunction with conventional treatment to ensure that your body is in the best possible state of health prior to starting ovulation induction or IVF. Your body will go into overdrive to produce between 8 to 12 eggs that month – potentially a whole year's supply! Your body needs to be in optimum condition so that when the embryo is implanted into your womb you have all the essential nutrients to ensure a successful pregnancy. Following a healthy diet and eliminating the 'nasty' toxins (smoking and drinking, etc.) will help you on your way.

Treatments like reflexology and acupuncture work well at balancing your internal energy systems while having treatment.

Some older women choose not to use conventional treatments to get pregnant and rely totally on improvements they have made to their diet and lifestyle to achieve conception.

Weight and fertility

Being the right body weight for pregnancy is very important. It sounds absurd to think that being too fat, too thin or exercising too much can affect your chances of getting pregnant, but it's true! Studies have found that very lean women and very obese women tend to have lower conception rates. It is not only being the right body weight that is critical for fertility – the amount of body fat you have is just as important. In normal adult women, fat comprises about 28 percent of body weight and, if it drops below 22 percent, then ovulation will stop. In addition, women with an average or above average body weight who exercise very rigorously may have a lower body fat and a higher muscle content, which also may lead to their periods becoming irregular or stopping altogether.

What about men? Weight loss or gain in men does affect their fertility, but not to the same degree as in women. The quality and quantity of sperm may be affected by severe weight loss through illness or anorexia. The production of the male sex hormone, testosterone, may decrease as a result of obesity, thus affecting fertility. Ideally, you and your partner should be healthy, active and following a preconception plan to increase your chances of having a baby.

Overweight and fertility

Being overweight can reduce your ability to conceive because it can affect your hormone levels and produce ovulatory problems. Obesity has a strong association with infertility and menstrual irregularities. Typically, being 20 percent over your ideal weight is considered obese. As an example, a 1.65 m (5ft 6in) woman weighing 72.45 kg (161 lb) has a BMI (body mass index) of 26 and is considered overweight. Losing 10 percent of her body weight or 7.2 kg (16 lb) would give her a new weight of 65.25 kg (145 lb) and a new BMI of 23.4, putting her in the normal weight range and increasing her chances of conception.

Being overweight increases the risk of pregnancy complications like miscarriage, gestational diabetes and pre-eclampsia. Women

Being overweight is such an important factor that a woman less than 30 years old with a BMI greater than 35 undergoing fertility treatment has about the same risk of miscarriage as a woman of normal weight who is over 40 years old.

with a BMI of between 30–35 (obese) have a miscarriage rate after fertility treatment of 27 percent, those with a BMI greater than 35 miscarry in 34 percent of cases.

Being overweight also adversely affects the outcome of fertility treatment. The success rate for IVF in obese women does not match that for women with a normal body mass.

Underweight and fertility

Being underweight also affects your fertility. Oestrogen levels fall and the menstrual cycle is affected; periods may even cease altogether (amenorrhoea). When a woman's percentage body fat falls below a certain minimum, her body does not produce the necessary levels of hormones to stimulate ovulation. She may be perfectly fertile, have plenty of healthy eggs in her body, yet her body does not release the eggs due to the lack of hormonal stimulation.

Many women are unnecessarily obsessed with their weight and may not realise the consequence of being too thin. It is one of the most common reasons for female infertility due to ovulation failure. A moderate weight loss of 10 to 15 percent under ideal body weight can result in menstrual irregularity and ovulation problems. Fifty percent of women who have a BMI of less than 20 stop ovulating and have fertility problems.

For example, the normal BMI range for a 1.65 m (5ft 6in) woman is 18.5–24.9, a body weight of between 51.3 kg (114 lb) and 69.3 kg (154 lb). Anything less than 51.3 kg (114 lb) would be underweight for this woman, and by gaining weight she would be improving her fertility. A group of underweight infertile women took part in a weight-gain programme and achieved 95 percent of their ideal body weights. This resulted in a spontaneous pregnancy rate of 73 percent.

What can I do?

If you are overweight Research has shown that a reduction of between 5 to 10 percent of your body weight increases fertility. Ideal ways of losing weight include changing to a healthy balanced diet and exercising three times per week. Ideally the exercise should include at least 20 minutes of cardiovascular exercise.

If you are unable to lose weight, investigate a potential illness. Many women are unable to lose weight despite diet and exercise plans. The additional weight is a side effect of an underlying illness. Conditions that can cause weight gain and obesity include PCOS (polycystic ovarian syndrome), an endocrine disorder resulting in irregular ovulation and Insulin Resistance Syndrome, which affects the body's ability to use insulin properly. If you are unable to lose weight through diet and exercise, it may be advisable to discuss your desire for having a baby with your doctor and to be evaluated for other conditions. Once these are brought under control, you may lose weight and subsequently increase your chances of conception.

If you are underweight Try and gain weight, in a healthy controlled way. It is not necessary to start eating burgers and chips to put on weight, just increase your portion size at every meal and maintain a healthy balanced diet as described in step 3. This will ensure you are eating all the essential vitamins and nutrients for conception. Monitor your menstrual cycle and see if you notice any changes, for example in the cervical mucus during ovulation and the length of your period as your weight increases.

So what is your ideal body weight?

BMI is a measurement of the relative percentages of fat and muscle mass in the human body. The measurement takes into account a person's weight and height to gauge total body fat. Medical professionals use the measurement as an indication of the risk of developing health problems such as heart disease and obesity. A BMI too high or too low affects fertility.

Body Mass Index is calculated as: weight (kg) / height (m) squared. For example, 65 kg / (1.72 m x 1.7 2m) = 65/2.95 = BMI of 22.03

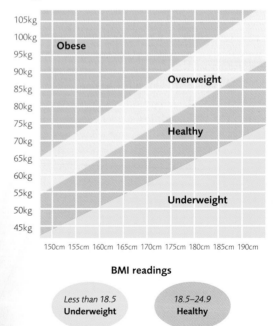

Weight		
105kg		
100kg	**Obese**	
95kg		
90kg		**Overweight**
85kg		
80kg		
75kg		**Healthy**
70kg		
65kg		
60kg		
55kg		**Underweight**
50kg		
45kg		

150cm 155cm 160cm 165cm 170cm 175cm 180cm 185cm 190cm

BMI readings

Less than 18.5	18.5–24.9
Underweight	**Healthy**

25.0–29.9	30–40	More than 40
Overweight	**Obese**	**Severely obese**

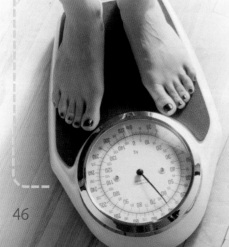

Lifestyle and fertility

Any book would not be complete without reviewing research and findings about how our lifestyle choices may affect our fertility. The last 10 years have seen a growth in evidence to support the fact that smoking, drinking, recreational drugs and certain environmental factors contribute to miscarriages, decreased sperm counts and infertility. You will know about many of the toxic chemicals discussed below, whereas others are more discrete and you may not be aware of their presence or the impact they may have on your fertility. In this section I aim to provide an overview of what the toxins are and how they specifically affect your fertility.

If, like me, you think that a few cups of tea or coffee a day, a little smoking when out with friends, and a few glasses of wine a week will not do you any harm, then read on. Aren't we told that everything in moderation is okay, a little of what you like is good for you? While I think this is true of many things, I certainly changed my mind when I read the mounting evidence presented to me. I decided if I was serious about conceiving a baby, the only way was to avoid any harmful chemicals that could put me and my baby-making chances at risk. While it is true that many of us know of someone who conceived while smoking and drinking, as I have learnt over the years, each person has different tolerance levels and what affects one person's body may not affect another's in the same way. Read the evidence below and draw your own conclusions. Only you will know what you consume and be able to judge if you should make any changes to your lifestyle during this important time.

Caffeine
Found in tea, coffee, cocoa, soft drinks, foods and medicines, caffeine primarily has a stimulating effect on the body. It can relieve fatigue, raise blood pressure and stimulate the kidneys. A normal cup of coffee contains about 90 mg of caffeine, tea contains 32 to 42mg of caffeine and cola drinks contain 16 mg in a 150 ml can. The stimulating effect of caffeine lasts between two-and-a-half to six hours.

Effect on women In 1980, a warning was issued by the US Food and Drug Administration advising pregnant women to restrict or eliminate drinking coffee given its ability to cause birth defects. Drinking coffee has been associated with reduced fertility. A study of 1,909 women found that drinking one cup of coffee per day increased their inability to get pregnant by 55 percent, for women drinking 2 to 3 cups per day this increased to 100 percent and for those who drank more than 3 cups per day, 176 percent higher. Coffee drinking before and during pregnancy doubled the risk of miscarriage if 2 to 3 cups per day were consumed. Drinking caffeine during pregnancy has been associated with chromosomal abnormality and late spontaneous abortion. It has been shown that after two cups of coffee, blood flow to the developing baby is significantly decreased, depriving it of essential oxygen and nutrients.

Effect on men Drinking moderate amounts of caffeine can affect sperm motility and large amounts can cause complete immobilisation of the sperm.

Cigarettes
Nicotine forms the major substance in cigarettes and is a highly addictive substance. Tobacco also contains over 4,000 other compounds including cyanide, carbon monoxide, lead, cadmium, ammonia and insecticides. The effect it has on reducing your chance of getting pregnant is well documented.

Effect on women Smokers have been shown to have an increased incidence of infertility, low birth-weight babies, miscarriages and stillbirths. Smokers are 3 to 4 times more likely than non-smokers to take more than a year to conceive. Smoking has a detrimental effect on the ovaries and research has shown that it accelerates the loss of eggs and may advance the advent of menopause, depending on how long a woman has smoked and the quantity. On average, babies born to mothers who smoked are 200 g (7 oz) lighter than those born to nonsmoking mothers. It is thought that cadmium, an inorganic poison present in smoke, becomes concentrated in the placenta while cyanide interferes with fetal nutrition, impeding growth. Smokers are more likely to produce eggs with genetic abnormalities, which increase the risk of miscarriage. Heavy smokers and drinkers have a six times greater risk of stillbirth as well as having babies born with malformations, including cleft palate, harelip and central nervous system abnormalities.

Effect on men Smokers have lower sperm counts, less active sperm and more abnormally shaped sperm. Again it is thought that the cadmium in tobacco is responsible and reduces the quality of the semen. Smokers' sperm counts are on average 13 to 17 percent lower than non-smokers. In one study, 42 percent of men who smoked suffered infertility compared to 28 percent in non-smokers.

Alcohol
It is now widely accepted that drinking alcohol has serious consequences on male sperm production and a woman's chances of conceiving, as well as harming the baby if consumed during pregnancy.

Alcohol has been proven to cause birth defects. Studies have tried to ascertain if a safe level may be consumed without causing any detrimental effects. Unfortunately, to date no substance which has been found to cause birth defects has an approved safe level of consumption. You should know that even moderate alcohol consumption (one to five drinks per week) has been associated with a decline in female fertility. In addition, it takes sperm 72 days to mature and the primary focus of the preconception plan is to avoid any toxins, including alcohol, three months before trying for a baby. Obviously, your aim is to have a healthy baby, free of any deformities, learning disabilities or illnesses.

Effect on women Research shows that children of alcohol-drinking mothers have lower IQs, signs of mental retardation, problems of the central nervous system, growth deficiencies, low birth weight, facial abnormalities and heart and dental defects. FAS (Fetal Alcohol Syndrome) is

now recognised as a condition in which children are born with abnormalities as a result of excess alcohol consumption during pregnancy. Consider this statement: 'The Fetal Alcohol Syndrome is now the third leading cause of mental retardation and neurological problems in infants, ranking after Down's syndrome and spina bifida' according to Dr. Noble of the National Institute of Alcohol Abuse and Alcoholism in the United States. The sad fact is these children may have been normal if the mother avoided alcohol during pregnancy.

Any drinking, even social, before or during pregnancy is a risk to your chances of conception and the growing of a healthy baby. In the first 21 days of fetal development, embryo cell division is taking place. If an excessive amount of alcohol is consumed before the embryo embeds into the uterus, the impact may be so severe that the baby is miscarried. Early miscarriages are common and often a woman may not even know she is pregnant; the only sign she may have of being pregnant is a delayed period. On day 36 of pregnancy essential parts of the baby are forming such as the limbs, brain, eyes, mouth and digestive tract. Alcohol consumed at this time can cause a defective heart, musculoskeletal abnormalities and mental handicap without any outward signs of FAS.

Effect on men Alcohol causes direct damage to the male reproductive organs such as the seminiferous tubules, which are responsible for sperm production. It is responsible for abnormal sperm, decrease in sperm quantity, sperm function and altered testosterone levels. It has been established that 80 percent of chronic alcoholic men are sterile and alcohol is one of the most common causes of male impotence.

Due to the severe outcome alcohol has on fertility, I can only recommend that both partners give up alcohol for at least three months before trying for a baby and maintain this throughout the duration of the pregnancy to ensure delivering a healthy baby nine months later.

Recreational drugs
Marijuana, cocaine and heroin also reduce your chance of getting pregnant.

Effect on women Recreational drugs interfere with the production of the female hormones, causing irregular or absent ovulation and periods. Cocaine increases the risk of the developing baby separating from the uterus in the third trimester, and that of stillbirth and heart defects. Heroin causes premature babies, stillbirths and growth deficiencies.

Effect on men Marijuana can lower levels of the male hormone, testosterone, reduce sperm counts and sperm motility and increase impotency. Heroin is known to lead to decreased fertility and deterioration of the male organs.

Psychology and fertility

It is widely accepted that infertility can trigger depression but can depression lead to infertility? New schools of thought suggest that psychological factors affecting fertility can be classified into two areas:
- Psychological factors that lead to infertility;
- Psychological distress resulting from the diagnosis and treatment of infertility.

The majority of infertile women report that infertility is the most upsetting experience of their lives. Research to date has primarily focused on the psychological distress following diagnosis. Depression associated with infertility is not the same as typical depression; it is a combination of emotions. You experience not just sadness but jealousy, anger and grief. Every month the woman is reminded once again that she has failed to become pregnant. It is a constantly recurring theme that seems endless.

Psychological factors that lead to infertility
The evidence suggests that depressive symptoms can have an adverse effect on the mind-body connection, thereby affecting fertility. Stress, anxiety and depression can alter immune function. We have all suffered from stress at some point and have subsequently become vulnerable to a cold or flu. When the body is run down, the visible symptom of the stress is revealed as a cold.

The internal effects of psychological stress and depression are harder to identify. Psychological factors affect the ability to get pregnant by: inhibiting or over-activating the hypothalamus, which helps to regulate hormonal levels; and altering pituitary gland functioning, which affects the hormonal balance necessary for ovulation, fertilisation, tubal functioning or even successful implantation of the egg once it reaches the womb.

Mood can have an effect on ovulation or embryo implantation, and high levels of stress may also cause fallopian tube spasm or decreased sperm production.

Research has shown that women suffering from depression, stress and anxiety are twice as likely to have problems conceiving. How many times have you heard stories of women who have fallen pregnant naturally just as they were about to embark on fertility treatment? Is this because they feel less under pressure now that the pregnancy outcome is in the hands of the experts? Have they suddenly become more fertile? Or has their outlook on the situation changed?

In one study, 60 percent of women who were treated for depression got pregnant within six months, as opposed to only 24 percent of untreated women. This suggests that once the symptoms of depression are cured, the body is more likely to conceive. Several studies conducted over the past three years support the theory that psychological distress can have a significant adverse impact on success rates in IVF.

Research on the mind-body connection is in its infancy; however, the evidence to date has been enlightening and provided some optimistic solutions for women suffering from depression.

Psychological distress following diagnosis and treatment
The psychological impact of infertility can be profound. It is reported that 10 percent of infertile women meet the criteria for a major depressive episode, 30–50 percent have depressive symptoms and 66 percent report feeling depressed after infertility treatment failure.

The incidence of depression and the severity of depressive episodes are higher in infertile

Environmental toxins

Many toxic elements are present in the air we breathe, the food we eat and the water we drink and can affect both male and female. Many toxins like lead have been known for years to cause harm to humans, whereas the effect of other environmental toxins has only just been discovered. A good example of this is the increased use of pesticides and herbicides by farmers in the last few decades. Nowadays supermarkets demand delicious healthy-looking fruit and vegetables at low prices, so farmers have little option but to use pesticides and herbicides to prolong shelf life and accentuate appearance. Some fruit and vegetables are sprayed 10 times before they reach the supermarket shelves, most of the residue of which is ingested by you. This is why eating organic food, which has avoided the intense spraying process, and drinking filtered or bottled water, significantly reduces the amount of environmental toxins you take in. Let's look at the most common environmental toxins affecting us today.

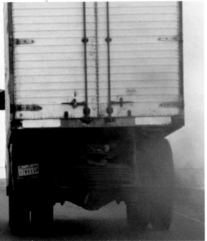

Lead is a highly toxic chemical found readily in the atmosphere, exhaust fumes and petrol. Over the years, regulations have come into place to reduce the amount of lead in our environment. Since 1960, all paint has been lead-free. Since 2000, leaded petrol has been phased out. Lead pipes found in older homes contaminate the water supply passing through them.

Lead affects both male and female reproductive capabilities. Men exposed to high levels of lead have a low sperm count and an increase in the number of abnormally shaped sperm. Women exposed to too much lead have high rates of infertility, miscarriage, stillbirth, and congenital abnormalities. To reduce your risk of ingesting lead, use unleaded petrol, drink filtered water and try to avoid busy, polluted roads where lead levels may be high.

Mercury has long been recognised as a poison despite being widely used in dentistry, pesticides and fungicides, and present in fish such as tuna. One study found female dentists to have a higher rate of miscarriage due to the daily handling of mercury. Nowadays dentists use white amalgam fillings and many offer a service to remove mercury fillings. Following my hair analysis results I chose to have my mercury fillings removed over a six-month period. My mouth seemed full of fillings, which I'm told do not cause much harm unless they leak mercury vapours. I have been known to grind my teeth at night and felt I would be happier if they were removed to avoid any chances of the mercury affecting my health.

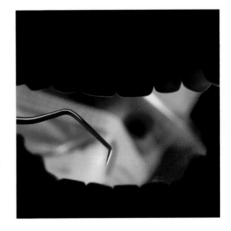

If you plan to have your fillings removed, do so a few months prior to trying to conceive, as vapour and fragments may be ingested as part of the removal process. The dentist should prescribe a 'detoxing'

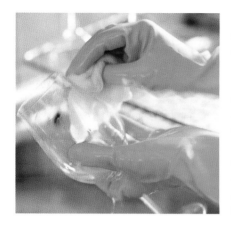

programme of supplements, which may include charcoal, multivitamins, selenium, vitamin C and plenty of water to minimise any side effect following removal.

Pesticides and herbicides are another set of toxic chemicals that have been found to have an adverse affect on our fertility. It seems that we cannot trust the quality of the food we eat any more. Food producers no longer have our best interests at heart; financial profit may be what drives them. For me this group of toxins are the most dangerous. Why? Because most of us do not know how many times the farmer has sprayed a toxic chemical onto the fruit to achieve the delicious looking appearance. Because it cannot be seen or smelt, it appears okay to eat. I was surprised to learn that pesticides are used in many everyday places like parks, gardens, lawns and golf courses; even British Rail spray the track and embankments with pesticides. They also are found in our water, DIY cupboards, carpets, wooden furniture and some medicines. One type of pesticide called organochlorine pesticides, contain a synthetic oestrogen. Studies have shown the use of this pesticide coincides with a decrease in sperm counts in the last decade, earlier onset of puberty in girls and an increase in the number of male babies born with problems with their genitals. While it is impossible to avoid daily exposure to low levels of pesticides, you can take certain measures to minimise your risk by choosing organic food, drinking filtered or bottled water and eating foods, which help eliminate toxic chemicals from the body (see below). Being aware of the problem is half the battle!

Peas and beans help mercury detoxification; eggs, butter, cold pressed oils (linseed oil, olive and sunflower) and citrus fruits help cleanse the liver; apples and pears, asparagus, Brussels sprouts and cabbage and garlic and onions, which are high in sulphur compounds, help remove mercury, cadmium and lead from the tissues. Additionally, nutritional supplements such as vitamins A, B complex and C, zinc and selenium, specifically assist in removing mercury and lead.

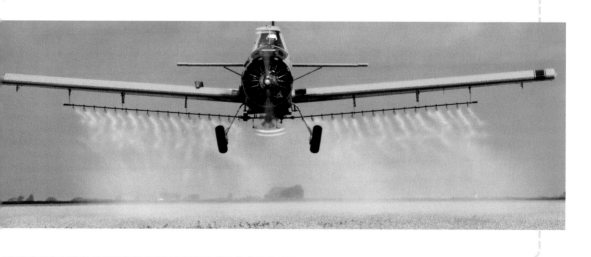

women than those in fertile couples. One study demonstrated that women dealing with infertility had the same levels of depression as women facing serious or life-threatening illnesses (like cancer). The only groups with a higher rate of depression were those women suffering from chronic-pain type illnesses.

There is a direct correlation between the length of infertility and occurrence of depression. Depression often occurs by the second to third year of infertility and does not return to normal levels until six years later.

Women who experienced depression following the failure of their first IVF, had much lower pregnancy rates than their non-depressed counterparts during their second IVF cycles.

One study reported that women who had a history of having taken antidepressants for more than six months were three times more likely to be infertile than women who had never taken antidepressants.

Treatment

Mind-body therapy The mind and body are inextricably linked. The mind governs thousands of processes, which enable us to function effectively. Treatments like hypnotherapy work on the premise that every thought or sensation experienced in the mind shows itself as some physical change in the body, and every physical change will have mental and emotional associations. The reproductive system is no exception. Mind-body treatment of infertility has been shown to both increase pregnancy rates as well as reducing psychological distress.

One study asked several hundred women with average infertility duration of 3.5 years to attend a mind-body programme centered on relaxation and other techniques. Forty-two percent conceived within six months of completing the program and there were significant decreases in all measured psychological symptoms including depression, anxiety and anger. The research does not stop there. Another study suggests that because mind-body programmes are effective for reducing negative emotions that may impair IVF success, patients should be offered such a programme in conjunction with IVF.

So is mind-body therapy more effective than counselling? One study set out to establish the most effective way to increase depressed infertile women's chances of conceiving. Women coping with infertility were placed into three different groups: a mind-body programme, a support group, or the control group, which received no support or relaxation advice. Fifty-five percent of the women in the mind-body programme went on to conceive, 54 percent of the women in the support group went on to conceive but only 20 percent of the women in the control group conceived. In other words, addressing the issue through mind-body therapy, hypnotherapy or counselling significantly increases the chance of pregnancy. Dealing with the issue is the key to success!

Counselling Many people do not seek the assistance of mental health services as they feel there is a social stigma associated with depression. Although physical conditions usually invoke sympathy in others, mention depression and the response is 'pull yourself together and get on with it'. I believe all infertile couples should be offered the services of fertility counsellors as part of the standard infertility treatment, even if they choose not to use it.

Support

Sometimes comfort and support can be found in the most unlikely places, such as chat rooms on the Internet. Many women like the anonymity of the forum and prefer to express their innermost thoughts and feelings to complete strangers. I set up my website, **www.3stepstofertility.com** exactly for that reason. The website is full of useful tips and information on infertility. More importantly, there is a forum for women to share stories and talk about their problems in the comfort of their own homes. Feel free to visit any time, who knows, you may feel better just talking about it!

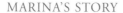

MARINA'S STORY

When I was diagnosed with infertility I kept myself incredibly busy researching, undergoing treatment and creating little projects for myself such as building a website, moving house and planning the next holiday. All the time I thought I was on top of the situation. It was not until I burst into tears one day in the supermarket over a simple gesture of motherly love – a woman caressed and gently kissed her baby girl while standing in the queue – that I realized how depressed I was about my infertility. I sobbed and sobbed, so much so, that I took to my bed for two days. I did not want to see anyone or speak to anyone; I wanted to be left alone! I had reached the depths of despair. The façade I portrayed to everyone including Simon had been convincing but inside I wanted to curl up in a corner and die. I could not cope anymore. I could not go on. How was I going to tell Simon I had had enough?

Each month I would cry alone in the bathroom when my period came and then have to pick myself up again to continue with life until the next month. Each time treatment failed Simon and I would retreat from our social engagements to avoid sympathetic looks from friends and family. Every time we had a setback we would console each other, often crying ourselves to sleep. We would say, 'At least we have each other, that's all that counts'. Over the years Simon and I became incredibly close, we are best friends, lovers and confidantes. However, despite the unconditional support we gave each other, I knew after five years something had to change; we could not live like this any longer.

One day my reflexologist gave me an article about infertile couples getting pregnant using hypnotherapy treatment. I immediately called the London clinic, curious to find out more about the mind-body connection and fertility. Within a week I started hypnotherapy sessions. Why? Something had to change and I was the only one who could break the downward spiral Simon and I were in. I had to change the way I looked at our situation. Over the years it had become a continuous cycle of optimism and excitement as we approached IVF treatment, followed by months of depression and emotional recovery preparing for the next attempt.

Hypnotherapy treatment is a powerful tool as it touches your innermost thoughts and feelings at a subconscious level. After five IVF attempts and being repeatedly told by doctors that my prospects of motherhood were slim, I had no confidence in myself, my body or my ability to get pregnant. Hypnotherapy helped erase those feelings of inadequacy, rebuild my confidence and, above all, showed me how powerful a positive mindset can be. It was so successful that I became pregnant naturally after ten sessions! The cloud had finally lifted; my outlook on life had changed forever. Despite miscarrying that pregnancy, I knew deep down I could become a mother after all. I am absolutely convinced that without the change in mindset I would have approached the last IVF attempt as before and Bruno would not be here today!

Depression is so debilitating to you and your life. My advice is to find a way to change your outlook by talking to friends, family and fertility counsellors or undergo hypnotherapy treatment – whatever it takes! Don't let your life pass you by; get out from under the cloud and take action now! A section in step 3 is dedicated to the benefits of hypnotherapy and how it may help you conceive.

AMY'S STORY

We conceived our first child within a couple of weeks of trying whilst on honeymoon without any regard for the optimum time for conception. We were exceptionally lucky as it just happened. Nine months later our son was born. Shortly before his second birthday we agreed that we would like to have another child. I had assumed that we were particularly fertile people and that, as with the first time, it would happen straight away. I remember the disappointment the first time my period arrived a few weeks later. After the second month without success I was even more disappointed but felt unable to share such feelings as I was only too aware of friends that had taken months, if not years, to conceive. I felt stupid and selfish for wanting to be pregnant so quickly. In today's consumer society if you decide you want something you can usually get hold of it, but nature is not so easily controlled. It was such a surprise not to be pregnant as for years we had taken so much care to prevent conception!

I was aware of friends who had used ovulation kits and purchased one myself. Despite having regular periods and a 26-day cycle I wasn't sure if I was ovulating at the middle of the month, as I had never experienced any pains or twinges that I had heard friends describe. We used the kits for a further few months but to no avail. In the end it actually had quite a damaging effect on our relationship in that neither of us liked the lack of spontaneity and felt under pressure to 'perform'. I would announce that the 'time was right' and if my husband wasn't immediately in the mood for action I would become upset. I discussed this with a girlfriend who suggested not making a declaration but when I tried this I felt like I was being deceptive and that didn't work either.

After six months we both agreed that enough was enough and we stopped using the ovulation kits. Instead, we agreed to relax and almost give up 'trying' as that clearly wasn't working. We tried to eat a healthy diet and cut down on alcohol. It was the New Year and we both felt quite unhealthy after the excesses of the festive season. Also my periods had gone from being regular to quite erratic for the first time in my life. During a visit to the local health-food shop a month or so later, I mentioned that I had been trying to conceive with a view to purchasing some folic acid. The saleswoman recommended that I should purchase some agnus castus to regulate my periods. She also recommended zinc tablets for me and my husband and suggested reflexology. I had heard that reflexology was quite relaxing and decided that it was probably nonsense but booked a session for the following week.

When I returned home I was quite sure that I had been ripped off and had been an easy mark, as I am quite sceptical about any form of alternative medicine. As I had purchased the products I decided I had better give them a go. I also attended the reflexology session and was utterly unconvinced and thought it was a complete waste of money! Six weeks later my period was late and I felt a little queasy. To my delight, I had a positive pregnancy test. It had taken almost 10 months to conceive but we had finally done it and we were thrilled. To this day I remain sceptical about the agnus castus, zinc and reflexology but perhaps it did help? I know that 10 months is really nothing but during that time I knew how my friends had felt when struggling to conceive for long periods and realized how much I had taken being pregnant for granted the first time around. It has made me appreciate and look forward to the birth of our second child so much more. I am due in three months' time and realise how lucky I am.

Secondary infertility

Secondary infertility is the inability to conceive another child after one or more successful pregnancies. WHO (the World Health Organisation) estimates that between 8 to 10 percent of couples suffer from infertility at some point in their lives; this equates to about 80 million people worldwide. In the UK, primary infertility occurs in 2.5 percent of women aged between 20 to 44 years old and secondary infertility in 9.9 percent of women. In other words, almost 4 times more couples have secondary infertility than primary infertility. This represented a staggering 1.6 million women in the UK in 1999.

Cause

The medical causes are similar to those of primary infertility and include tubal disease, ovulation difficulties, endometriosis, and sperm dysfunction. However, there are differences. It is thought that age plays a significant factor in secondary infertility, as the couple are now older when trying to conceive for the second time. Other theories include the possibility of stress and lifestyle changes affecting the couple's fertility. Looking after the first child and enduring sleepless nights, and the additional workload and stress of parenthood all can impact on a couple's ability the second time around. There simply just may not be enough time in the day!

Seeking a solution

As with primary infertility, a step-by-step approach is recommended for getting to the bottom of the problem.

The first step is to understand what may be affecting your fertility. What has changed since you last conceived? Is your lifestyle different in any way? Are you overweight? Have you lost too much weight chasing around after your first child? Are you juggling a job and motherhood? Is your partner stressed at work? Are you feeling stressed? Are you eating properly? Are you happy in your relationship? Have you been ill? Are you recovering from an illness? Did you have a difficult first childbirth? Did you/do you have postnatal depression? All these factors could be

Emotional aspects

Couples with secondary infertility may find it difficult to gain the same level of sympathy and encouragement from family and friends as couples with primary infertility. In some ways they are the envy of couples with primary infertility, who view them as 'lucky to have one child' while fertile couples cannot understand why they are having problems conceiving a second child if they've already had one child. Thus couples with secondary infertility are caught between the worlds of the infertile and fertile!

As time passes, the frustration can be intolerable. Many couples specify a particular time to conceive a second child, 'when little David is two years old would be ideal' yet when the time comes, it does not happen for whatever reason. Suddenly the couple questions their ability to conceive and for the first time start researching what they can do to help themselves. Unfortunately, being pregnant once doesn't make them immune to all the conditions that can cause infertility.

having an effect on your ability to conceive for the second time. Stop and take time to evaluate how you and your partner are feeling and be honest with yourselves. Trying to conceive another child while looking after one child is not easy and it may be taking its toll on you without you realising the consequences.

If after the review the reason becomes apparent to you both, take action to address the issue. The most positive way forward is to identify what the problem is and make the necessary changes, be it to your diet, your home life, job or relationship, and then keep trying!

Secondly, you should complete the fertility tests. If after you have both reviewed your situation and there is no obvious reason why you and you partner are having difficulty, it is worth commencing fertility investigations. Arrange an appointment with your doctor to commence testing. Details of the tests performed can be found in step 2. If, after testing, a reason for your infertility is discovered, it means you can review the treatment options available to you and progress to the next stage.

Finally, research and review all the complementary and conventional treatments discussed in step 3 and discuss the options with your doctor. Once you have chosen the best way forward, start the preconception wholefood diet to ensure your body is in peak condition to get pregnant and carry a baby to full term.

Essentially the three steps to fertility, the subject of this book, is a process designed for couples experiencing both primary and secondary infertility, as the causes and methods of treatment are the same for both. The ultimate goal is to get pregnant and deliver a healthy baby into this world!

Treatment

This follows the same path as primary fertility. Female fertility tests focus on hormonal and structural aspects of the reproductive system. The male tests analyze the quality and quantity of sperm. The cause of infertility may be identified and the doctor will discuss treatment options with you. Research has shown that couples with secondary infertility are more likely to achieve a second pregnancy, even with conventional methods like IVF.

Complementary treatments like reflexology and acupuncture will re-balance the energy meridians and encourage relaxation. The advice on diet remains the same for secondary infertility – eat all the essential vitamins and minerals in abundance! Take time out with just you and your partner, away from the daily routine of parenting and work.

What can go wrong?

It would be negligent of me to discuss all the positive aspects of preparing for pregnancy without discussing the reality of what can go wrong when you do become pregnant or undergo fertility treatment. The three most common problems are:
- Miscarriage and recurrent miscarriage
- Ectopic pregnancy
- OHSS (ovarian hyperstimulation syndrome)

Each one has a devastating effect on a couple: with miscarriage, conception has taken place but the fetus has failed to develop normally; with ectopic pregnancy, conception has taken place but in the wrong place and, finally, with OHSS, following her IVF treatment, a woman's body is unable to receive a healthy fertilized embryo as she is too ill. All these conditions are heart-breaking. Most of us work hard to get pregnant by whatever means and may have thought we had overcome all the obstacles. Then, wham! Another blow to deal with! The 'infertile' umbrella does not just include women who have problems getting pregnant, it also encompasses women who do not carry a baby to full term, e.g. have suffered a miscarriage or ectopic pregnancy. In both cases, the body is saying it can create an embryo but there are other underlying reasons why the embryo does not grow to full term.

Miscarriage

One in four women have at least one miscarriage – around a quarter of a million women in the UK each year. Recurrent miscarriage (defined as three consecutive miscarriages) affects approximately one percent of women.

Causes

Miscarriage can be a result of genetic, hormonal, immunological, physiological, anatomical or environmental factors.

Genetic problems Early pregnancy loss (before 12 weeks) is associated with chromosomal abnormalities in 50 to 60 percent of cases. As women age, miscarriage becomes more common partly due to the quality of the eggs diminishing. At age 35 to 39 years, a woman has a 21 percent chance of miscarriage compared to 42 percent if she is over 42 years of age.

Hormonal Women with very irregular periods may find it harder to conceive and when they do, are more likely to miscarry.

Immunological The study of immunology in relation to infertility, pregnancy and miscarriage is still relatively new and more research is needed until it is fully understood. The treatments available may be controversial and schools of thought differ in their opinions of their efficacy. Many doctors recommend a comprehensive blood test to assess the presence of cytokines, natural killer cells, antiphospholipids and thrombophilia, especially if a woman suffers recurrent pregnancy loss. Experts in the field of immunology categorise the cause of the loss into three categories.

Implantation loss occurs more frequently than we know. The sperm and egg have fertilised successfully, however the embryo fails to implant in the uterus. It is thought that up to 40 percent of embryos are lost at around the time of implantation. Some women may briefly 'feel' pregnant, only to find their period begins a few weeks later. Women with unexplained infertility, implantation failure after IVF or women with a family history of autoimmune diseases like lupus may have a blood test to test for the presence of cytokines and antiphospholipids. An embryo grows to approximately 3 mm two weeks after fertilisation and can receive adequate blood supply. As it continues to grow it is thought additional blood vessels are needed to keep up with demand. Studies have shown that cytokines and antiphospholipids play a role in the development of these vital blood vessels. Lack of development would cause blood clotting and prevent the embryo receiving an adequate blood supply.

Early pregnancy losses are losses of embryos during the first trimester of pregnancy. Early and late pregnancy losses are thought to occur for a

different reason to implantation loss. During the first trimester a blood supply between the mother and baby has been established. Pregnancy loss during the first and second trimester may be due to an interference of the blood supply to the developing baby. Research has shown that women suffering a late pregnancy loss have a high incidence of thrombophilia. A blood test can determine if the cause is genetic.

Chromosome abnormalities still account for the majority of reasons why a pregnancy is lost at this stage and further research is needed.

Infection Minor infections like coughs and colds are not harmful, but a very high temperature and some illnesses, such as German measles, may cause miscarriage. The role of vaginal infections in the causation of miscarriage is being researched further.

Anatomical If the cervix (neck of the womb) is weak, it may start to open as the uterus (womb) becomes heavier in later pregnancy (beyond 14 weeks) and this may lead to miscarriage. The insertion of a cervical stitch is often recommended. An irregular-shaped uterus can mean that there is not enough room for the baby to grow. It is estimated that this represents up to 10 percent of women who repeatedly miscarry. Large fibroids may cause miscarriage in later pregnancy.

Environmental Women who smoke have an increased risk of miscarriage, as do women with excessive alcohol intakes.

Recurrent Miscarriages

It is thought that other factors, in addition to those above, play a role in recurrent miscarriages. Recent research has shown blood-clotting disorders to be linked to recurrent miscarriages. Blood thickens during pregnancy and if clots occur in the blood vessels of the placenta, the baby will not receive an adequate supply to develop normally. A woman may be tested for the antibody – APA (antiphospholipid antibody) – that causes blood to clot more easily. Reports show that 15 percent of women with recurrent miscarriages have tested positive for

JULIE'S STORY

Jack was 18 months old and we were ready for another baby. It had taken a year to conceive first time and I thought it might be the same this time, but in my first month off the pill, baby number two was on his way, or so we thought!

The first twelve weeks passed and I nervously looked forward to my first scan date. On several occasions I protested to my mum that I didn't even feel pregnant, yet as I was certainly thickening round the waist, it could have been something to do with the frenzied eating!

Just before the scan was due I woke suddenly and felt like I had gone into labour. Within minutes I felt a tell-tale warm feeling in the nether regions. After visiting the toilet and confirming I was bleeding I got straight on line to find out every gory detail about the unspoken fear: miscarriage. I spent hours avidly reading with tears streaming down my face – I had learnt everything there is about miscarriage. One of the hardest moments was sharing the fear with my parents, who were devastated by what might be bad news for Bob and me.

In the morning we had a scan; the radiographer confirmed there was no heartbeat. We were devastated. I had suffered a missed miscarriage and the baby had died at seven weeks but my body had not expelled it until 12 weeks. My dad, a tough northerner, 'wept buckets' my mum told me afterwards. You don't really think about the effect a miscarriage has on the wider family but clearly the loss of a future grandchild was equally devastating to my parents. Suddenly all the expectation and plans Bob and I had made disappeared in an instant.

Three months later I was pregnant again and nervous from the start. At six weeks I couldn't believe it was happening again! I had read the statistics about miscarriages but I was going to be lucky this time, surely! The pregnancy was confirmed as a blighted ovum; no baby had ever existed. I was heartbroken!

I agonized over trying again but four months after my second heartbreak I was pregnant again. I didn't experience any pregnancy symptoms and my daily mantra was 'please let it be okay'. At my 12-week scan a healthy pregnancy was confirmed; what a relief, yet I still did not relax fully until about 20 weeks. In May of this year my little angel, Eve, was born. I sobbed not only with happiness when she was born, but utter relief that she was here! My friends will tell you that religion is not central to my life but Eve is my little gift from God.

I admit I stretched the truth when seeing a specialist about the causes of my miscarriages; I said I had had three miscarriages, not two! Apparently detailed investigations only take place if a woman has suffered three miscarriages. I couldn't bear going through another pregnancy loss again to find out why it was happening.

The specialist was great; he told me nature is the best judge of a baby's survival chances and it decides very early on whether a baby is viable. My first loss was due to nature knowing something the medical people didn't. It allowed my baby to slip away because his chances of survival were slim. With the second loss, the baby never actually existed, though the devastation was the same. The specialist made me understand that in 90 percent of cases it is the result of a hormone imbalance and somehow you have to get your head around that!

APA. Aspirin and heparin thin the blood. Women given aspirin had a 40 percent success rate compared to 70 percent success rate when both aspirin and heparin were taken.

For more information on the connection between infertility, miscarriages and immunology visit www.repro-med.net and www.haveababy.com. Each website deals with the new findings and research in detail.

Ectopic pregnancy

This is a pregnancy where the fetus develops outside the uterus. Most commonly it develops in the fallopian tube. Other less common sites are the abdominal cavity and ovaries. Tubal pregnancy occurs in 1 in 200 pregnancies. If the pregnancy ends early and the embryo is reabsorbed, the only sign of the miscarriage having occurred is a delayed period. On the other hand, if the embryo continues to grow within the fallopian tubes, it may lead to a rupturing of the tube between the 10th and 14th week. The rupture may happen slowly over a few weeks or suddenly burst, causing internal bleeding. This condition is life threatening for the mother, and the embryo (and usually the tube) is removed as a matter of urgency.

Cause

There are many factors that increase the risk of ectopic pregnancy:

- Salpingitis – an infection of the fallopian tubes;
- PID (pelvic inflammatory disease) can cause damage to the fine hairs, cilia, that waft the embryo towards the uterus;
- Fibroids – pressure on the tube may lead to obstruction;
- Endometriosis;
- Progesterone-only pills (the mini pill), as they inhibit the milking action of the fallopian tubes, which transfers the egg to the uterus;
- Surgery of the fallopian tube or reverse tubal sterilisation.

Symptoms

A pregnant women may be experiencing the normal symptoms of pregnancy – morning sickness and tenderness of the breast – and be totally unaware of the tubal pregnancy. Spotting, passing of clots and a dull ache in the abdomen may occur. If the tube ruptures, the pain is usually sudden and sharp. Internal bleeding leads to nausea, fainting, hot and cold sweats and an increased irregular pulse rate.

Diagnosis

Because many of the symptoms are the same as early miscarriage or a 'threatened miscarriage' – abdominal pain and/or bleeding – diagnosis is incredibly difficult and an ectopic pregnancy may not be detected until the tube has ruptured. As soon as any symptoms appear, visit the doctor, who will perform a blood test to confirm the pregnancy. If the blood test is positive and you are more than six weeks' pregnant, an ultrasound scan will show no fetus in the uterus if the pregnancy is ectopic. If the symptoms appear before six weeks it is difficult to see the baby on the scan, so the doctor may perform a blood test over the following few days. If the human growth hormone levels increase each day, it confirms a baby is developing within your body but not in the uterus. If the hormone levels do not increase each day, it confirms that the baby has died and the bleeding may be the signs of miscarriage.

Treatment

Surgery is performed as soon as it is confirmed the pregnancy is ectopic as it is a life-threatening condition. In most cases when the fallopian tube ruptures, it is surgically removed with the fetus. Before the operation, it is important to talk through all the options with the surgeon, especially if you want to try for a baby again. Doctors are very sympathetic to the situation and will ensure that as much as possible of the reproductive capabilities are preserved.

OHSS (Ovarian Hyperstimulation Syndrome)

This is a complication of controlled ovarian stimulation arising in approximately five percent of women undergoing fertility treatment. Ovulation induction uses drugs containing gonadotrophins, which mimic the production of the natural female hormones. The side effect of the fertility drug is ovarian hyperstimulation syndrome. Some women are more susceptible – those with polycystic ovarian syndrome, younger women and women with previous OHSS are more sensitive to the fertility drugs than others. Essentially the fertility drugs are encouraging the body to produce the right amount of follicles and eggs. Ideally seven to 12 eggs may be collected from among 10 to 20 follicles. In OHSS, the body may overproduce follicles. Egg collection still takes place but rather than embryos being put back into the uterus, they are all frozen until you have recovered from the overstimulation, which usually takes a few weeks. Live embryos produce higher success rates than frozen eggs or embryos, so the success rate is reduced from

25 percent to 10 percent on average. In 2003, in 75 percent of cases of IVF, women used fresh embryos from their own eggs, 19 percent used frozen embryos from their own eggs and the remaining six percent used donor eggs.

A diagnosis of OHSS is devastating news. The woman has spent the last few weeks mentally preparing herself for the egg transfer process and as a result of OHSS; she goes home 'empty'. Mild and moderate forms of OHSS occur in approximately five percent of women undergoing ovulation induction treatment; one percent suffers the more severe form. Symptoms begin to appear four to five days after the egg collection. If pregnancy occurs, the symptoms can worsen as the body's natural HCG (human chorionic gonadotrophin) increases as a result of pregnancy. If signs of OHSS are apparent prior to embryo transfer, the consultant may not proceed with the treatment and preserve the embryos until a later date by freezing (cryopreservation).

Prevention

Each clinic in the UK provides patients with information about the risk of OHSS following ovulation induction treatments. The best prevention is to bring the condition to a patient's attention, explaining what symptoms to look for

The severity of symptoms and their treatment		
Mild	Ovarian enlargement, slight abdominal pain and swelling, diarrhoea.	Pain relief. Drink plenty of water. Refrain from strenuous activity.
Moderate	Noticeable pain and bloating, nausea and vomiting, breathing difficulties, faintness, dehydration, thirstiness, weight gain, clothes feel tight, dark urine.	Pain relief, lots of water, bed rest. You may be monitored daily by the doctor to ensure symptoms do not worsen.
Severe	Can lead to leakage of hormones and fluid from the ovaries, causing accumulation of fluid in abdominal cavity and chest. Marked abdominal distension, shortness of breath, pain in calf and chest, heart attack or stroke, kidney damage.	Hospital admission to remove the excess fluid from the abdominal cavity, re-balance fluid and electrolytes. Usually feel better within 7–10 days.

and the problems that may occur, in order to increase her awareness. Many women do not know they are sensitive to the effects of fertility drugs until it is too late.

Throughout the fertility treatment, the clinic will carefully monitor your progress with ultrasound scans and blood tests to measure high oestrogen levels. At any time, if it appears the woman's body is showing signs of OHSS, the consultant may advise 'coasting' – stopping the gonadotrophin stimulation until oestrogen levels decline to acceptable levels before proceeding to egg collection. There is a very fine line between stimulating the ovaries just enough to collect sufficient eggs, to the body going into overdrive and overstimulating. The main advice is to follow the preventative advice to the letter, even if you find it difficult. It will pay huge dividends as it's the difference between having a live embryo transfer or not. You will be maximising your chances if you do so!

ULTRASOUND MONITORING
This is required to keep track of the developing follicles.

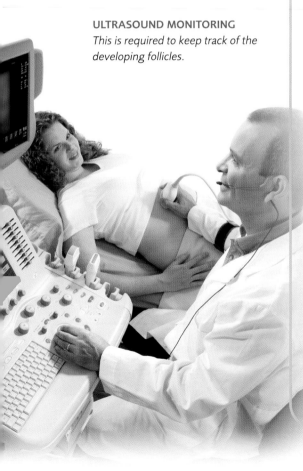

MARINA'S STORY

Having suffered from moderate OHSS twice, my advice is do all that you can to prevent it happening. It is disheartening to be told at the last hurdle that the fertilised embryos will be frozen, as you are too unwell for embryo transfer. As we progressed towards embryo transfer day, our excitement grew; it all seemed to be going so well UNTIL about three days before. Poor Simon had to sit by while his hopes of fatherhood were taken away from him because I was too sick. He was incredibly understanding but I still couldn't help feeling I had let him down.

The first time I was unaware of my susceptibility to OHSS. The second time, despite preventative measures, I was even more sensitive to the fertility drugs. The situation was made worse because that clinic coasted me over a holiday weekend.

Throughout my last IVF cycle I was very anxious about how the clinic would manage overstimulation if it occurred. I desperately wanted to have a live embryo transfer as I knew it was my best chance of success. During the 10 days prior to egg collection, I visited the clinic every morning and afternoon for an oestrogen blood test and ultrasound scan. Each night I received a call from the consultant telling me how much hormone to administer the following day. I was being monitored extremely closely to ensure my body did not suddenly overreact to the fertility drugs. The IVF programme was completely tailored to my needs, unlike previous attempts. I was advised to drink four litres of water a day and ½ litre of milk – that's about 17 glasses a day! I felt like a human fountain and was constantly on the toilet but it worked! For the first time I had a live embryo transfer and I became pregnant with Bruno!

Are you ready for pregnancy?

Section A **Background**	Female	Male

Height (m)

Weight (kg)

	Female		Male	
Are you underweight (BMI less than 18.5)?	○ Yes	○ No	○ Yes	○ No
Are you overweight (BMI over 25)?	○ Yes	○ No	○ Yes	○ No

Body Mass Index (BMI) (weight (kg) divide by height (m) squared
(e.g. 65 kg / (1.72 x 1.72) = 65/2.95 =22.03)

Section B **Diet**		

	Female		Male	
Do you drink caffeine/caffeinated drinks?	○ Yes	○ No	○ Yes	○ No
How many per day?				
Do you smoke cigarettes?	○ Yes	○ No	○ Yes	○ No
How many per day?				
Alcohol units consumed per week?				
Do you use recreational drugs?	○ Yes	○ No	○ Yes	○ No
Which best describes your diet?	**A, B** or **C?**		**A, B** or **C?**	

A

Breakfast: fried egg on toast, muffin, tea/coffee.

Lunch: Pizza and chips.

Dinner: Curry with white rice and vegetables, wine/beer. Ice cream.

Snacks: chocolate, cake and biscuits.

2 glasses water, 3 teas, 1 coke/lemonade.

B

Breakfast: Grain cereal, juice, fruit.

Lunch: Grilled chicken and salad.

Dinner: Fish, brown rice and steamed vegetables, fruit, mostly organic produce.

Snacks: Fruit and vegetables, seeds, raisins, etc.

Eight glasses water per day.

C

combination of both A and B

Section C **Lifestyle**	Female	Male

Stress factor (on scale of 1–10)

How many hours do you work per week?

How many hours do you sleep per night?

How many times do you make love per month?

How many times do you exercise per week?

	Female		Male	
Do you work with chemicals?	○ Yes	○ No	○ Yes	○ No
Do you have high blood pressure?	○ Yes	○ No	○ Yes	○ No

Section D **Female history**

Have you suffered from any of the following in the past or currently? (Tick box[es])

- ◯ Irregular periods
- ◯ No periods
- ◯ Low back pain
- ◯ Ovulation pain
- ◯ Pain on intercourse
- ◯ Painful periods

- ◯ Premenstrual tension
- ◯ Thrush
- ◯ Vaginal discharge
- ◯ Cystitis
- ◯ Fibroids
- ◯ Endometriosis

- ◯ Ovarian cysts
- ◯ Genital warts
- ◯ Gonorrhoea
- ◯ Chlamydia
- ◯ Syphilis
- ◯ Herpes

- ◯ AIDS
- ◯ Miscarriage
- ◯ Ectopic pregnancy
- ◯ Stillbirth

Section E **Male history**

Have you suffered from any of the following in the past or currently? (Tick box[es])

- ◯ Erectile dysfunction
- ◯ Ejaculation problems
- ◯ Testicular injury (sport)
- ◯ Undescended testes
- ◯ Hernia
- ◯ Mumps

- ◯ Chlamydia
- ◯ Herpes
- ◯ AIDS
- ◯ Gonorrhoea
- ◯ Syphilis

Do you regularly:

Soak in hot baths?	◯ Yes	◯ No
Have saunas/jacuzzis?	◯ Yes	◯ No
Work in high environmental temperatures?	◯ Yes	◯ No
Wear tight underwear?	◯ Yes	◯ No
Sit for long periods of time? (e.g. travelling salesman/lorry driver)	◯ Yes	◯ No

Section F **Emotional assessment**

	Female		Male	
Are you happy in your relationship?	◯ Yes	◯ No	◯ Yes	◯ No
Do you have any fears about pregnancy?	◯ Yes	◯ No	◯ Yes	◯ No
Do you have any fears about fetal abnormalities?	◯ Yes	◯ No	◯ Yes	◯ No
Do you have any fears about childbirth?	◯ Yes	◯ No	◯ Yes	◯ No
Do you have any fears about becoming a parent?	◯ Yes	◯ No	◯ Yes	◯ No
Are you worried how you will cope?	◯ Yes	◯ No	◯ Yes	◯ No
Are you worried how your career may be affected?	◯ Yes	◯ No	◯ Yes	◯ No
Are you worried about your financial situation?	◯ Yes	◯ No	◯ Yes	◯ No
Are you worried you are too old?	◯ Yes	◯ No	◯ Yes	◯ No

Section G **Pre-conception preparation**

Have you stopped taking contraception?	◯ Yes	◯ No
Taking an antenatal vitamin supplement and folic acid?	◯ Yes	◯ No
Tracking ovulation (Billings method or ovulation testing kits)?	◯ Yes	◯ No
Actively having sex several times during ovulation?	◯ Yes	◯ No

Your answers explained

SECTION A

Body Mass Index is a measurement of the relative percentages of fat and muscle mass in the human body and the result is used as an index of obesity. Being the right weight is important for fertility. Being underweight can cause oestrogen levels to fall and periods may become intermittent or stop altogether. Being overweight can also affect hormonal balance and prevent ovulation.

The ranges are:

Underweight	less than 18.5
Normal	18.5–24.9
Overweight	25.0–29.9
Obese	greater than 30
Extreme obesity	over 40

If you are underweight you need to gain weight, if you are overweight you will maximise your chances of conceiving by losing weight. Following the wholefood programme will help you to lose weight and ensure you include all the essential nutrients for conception.

SECTION B

If you answered 'yes' to any of the questions you are putting harmful toxins into your body, which will affect fertility. To maximise your chances, cut them out!

Diet A – help!
This diet has insufficient vitamins and minerals and is full of empty calories. You will need to dramatically modify your diet to include foodstuffs, which are missing and eliminate caffeine. The wholefood diet will help you with your choices.

Diet B – well done!
You are eating a healthy balanced diet full of nourishment for conception.

Diet C – You are halfway there!
Slight adjustments will be needed if you want to be in optimum health for conception and pregnancy.

SECTION C

Stress factor
Less than 5 - you have a relaxed outlook on life and take life's challenges in your stride. Continue the good work!

Between 5 and 7 you have moments of stress in your life but find ways of managing them when they arise and do not let it adversely affect your health. For those moments, take time out, go to the gym, relax and unwind!

Greater than 7 indicates that you operate at a stressed level most of the time and find it difficult to cope. You may resort to smoking and drinking to calm you down and eat on the go! Your fertility is affected as stress interferes with hormone production and blood flow to the reproductive organs. Finding ways to relax is key to decreasing your stress levels. Treatments like reflexology can help to calm your mind and relax your body. Massage and deep-breathing exercises may help to reduce the tension in your body.

Having the right work-life balance is important when trying for a baby. Long hours and lack of quality sleep may cause you to feel tired, run down and lethargic. Making love may be the last thing on your mind and having to rise to the occasion several times over a three-day period can put additional strain on your body and relationship that would otherwise not be a problem if you were feeling relaxed and stress free. Make sure you find time to relax.

SECTION D AND E

If you have ticked any of the boxes relating to previous illnesses or current symptoms you will need to visit your GP for further tests. Details of the routine fertility tests performed are discussed in step 2.

SECTION F

If you have circled 'yes' to any of the statements it is worth assessing how mentally prepared you are for a baby. Often, deep-rooted fears and worries can accumulate in your mind to such an extent that it prevents conception taking place. You and your partner should address any issues prior to trying for a baby. Many support groups exist specifically to assist infertile couples to deal with infertility, details of these groups can be found in the appendix. Family and friends are also a great source of support as they have your best interests at heart.

SECTION G

If you answered 'yes' to all the questions – well done! You are taking all the right actions to prepare your body for pregnancy. Doctor's surgeries now widely advertise the benefits of taking folic acid up to three months before conceiving to prevent conditions like spina bifida. Many antenatal vitamins can be bought from pharmacies, which combine all the essential vitamins and minerals in one tablet. Ovulation kits are available to help you identify when you are ovulating each month. With all the information, supplements and tools readily available, it is easier than ever before to maximise your chances of conception.

Summary

We have now come to the end of this chapter on understanding your body. You may be discouraged by the amount of information about infertility. You may be asking yourself, 'Do I really need to know about every aspect of my body and infertility to improve my chances of getting pregnant?'. The honest answer is, 'Yes'. You need to know enough to be at ease when discussing your situation with the medical professionals. You need to be able to translate the terminology, delve into possible causes and evaluate your options without apprehension and ambiguity. Only you will know how much information that is!

Without a doubt it can be disheartening reviewing the causes of infertility and, especially, what can go wrong if you do become pregnant. It may seem like there are too many obstacles to overcome – it will never happen! Rest assured, gaining knowledge about infertility, the good and the bad, and becoming your own expert, will empower you and make you feel more confident about the process. Fertility specialists will guide you but no one cares as much about your fertility and getting pregnant as you do – research, question and above all remain positive!

Many women have written stories about their own personal experiences to help, inspire, support and comfort you. We want you to feel determined and hopeful in your quest to have a baby. With that in mind, it is time to move onto step 2 – completing the necessary fertility tests.

step 2

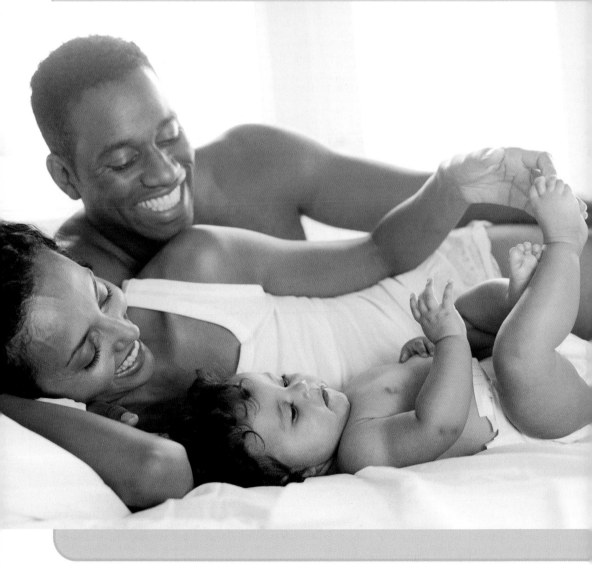

Complete the tests

The second step to fertility is to complete all necessary tests to identify the reason(s) for infertility. Fertility tests are designed to uncover hormonal and structural problems in both partners.

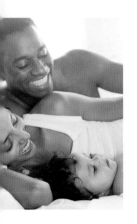

Before I delve into the tests, I would like to say 'well done' to you for getting this far. It is not easy to actively try for a baby for a year and then come to the realisation that there may be something wrong. Your relationship may be feeling the strain and both of you are probably praying that you're not the one with the problem. Emotions will be running at an all-time high; you're happy that a reason may be discovered as to why conception hasn't happened, but you'll be nervous and anxious about what the tests will reveal. I hope I can ease some of your difficulties by providing you with insights into why the tests are performed, what you can expect from them, and what they can show.

Why is fertility testing so important?

There are a couple of very important reasons for having your fertility tested. The first is that it identifies the cause of your inability to conceive and the second is that it prevents unnecessary treatment.

Being able to identify the cause of your infertility and giving it a name can be an enormous relief for a couple. It enables you to move forward and start exploring potential treatments. You are one step closer to maximising your chances of conception. I won't deny the fact that the process of investigating infertility can be humiliating, embarrassing, invasive and demoralising but, on the positive side, you will know what is wrong!

Try and work through the tests one at a time. It is difficult to know how you will feel or react to the situation. Some people are very matter of fact about the process; others become filled with fear and trepidation.

I have seen cases where couples rush in and opt for in vitro fertilisation (IVF) without truly understanding if their problem is hormonal, structural, a combination of issues or can be resolved simply with nutritional and other lifestyle changes. All they want is a baby at any cost and right now! Undergoing fertility treatment often puts additional emotional, physical and financial strain on the individual and his or her relationship, which could otherwise be avoided if the true cause of the infertility was known beforehand.

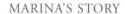

MARINA'S STORY

My husband, Simon, and I muddled our way through the fertility testing stage. I found it difficult to come to terms with the fact that having a baby would not come naturally to me and refused to talk about it to anyone apart from Simon for the first two years. Simon was sworn to secrecy and, if at any stage I thought someone else knew I was a failure, an argument ensued! We lived in this little bubble of our own making. I finally emerged from my bubble and told our family and closest friends what we had been through. By that time I had been diagnosed with endometriosis, faulty fallopian tubes and had completed two IVF attempts. I was astounded by everyone's compassion and support. Suddenly we realised that we didn't need to deal with our issue on our own and we had missed out on the best support group available – those people around us that care!

What should I do first?

If you and your partner have been actively having sex and made the necessary recommended dietary and lifestyle changes (see pages 47–9) for over a year, you should make an appointment with your doctor to start investigating the potential reasons why you have not yet conceived. However, if you have just started trying for a baby (three to six months) and are under 35 years old, it is wise to embark on a period of healthy living prior to visiting a doctor. Your body may just need a period of cleansing and a nutritional boost in order to achieve conception. By trying a natural approach first, you may avoid unnecessary investigations, which can cause stress between partners and may add to your infertility problems.

Following your appointment with your doctor, you may be referred to a specialist who will ask both of you to provide a detailed sexual and medical history before taking blood samples for hormonal assessment.

Your doctor and/or specialist may perform some or all of the tests outlined right. Finding the cause of infertility is essentially a process of elimination; once the problem is identified, you will progress to the next stage – choosing the right treatment. Not all women will need to have an internal examination. If, for example, it becomes evident that the woman has hormonal issues and her partner a reduced sperm count, you will progress to starting recommended treatments for these problems.

I discuss the tests in the sequence your doctor and/or gynaecologist should perform them. It makes sense to carry out invasive tests like a laparoscopy only when all the blood and hormone tests have come back showing that your hormones are not to blame.

Allow at least two to three months for fertility testing. Some tests are taken at specific times of the monthly cycle (see page 76) and others may require booking in advance so you can take time off work.

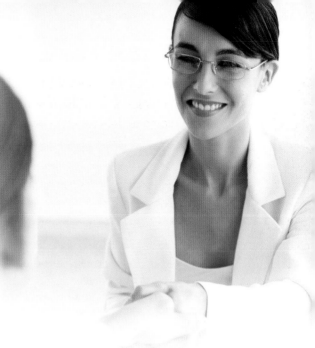

Common fertility tests

Both partners

Details of medical history

HIV

Hepatitis B & C

STDs – Syphilis/ Gonorrhoea/Chlamydia

Genetic screening if family history i.e. cystic fibrosis

Male	Female
Semen analysis	Basal Body Temperature (BBT)
	Rubella
Hormone tests	Rhesus test
	Luteinising hormone (LH)
	Follicle stimulating hormone (FSH)
	Oestradiol
	Progesterone
	Post Coital Test (PCT)
	Ultrasound
	Hystersalpingogram(HSG)
	Laparoscopy
	Hysteroscopy
	Endometrial biopsy
	Autoimmune testing

Tests for both partners

Typically a doctor will start by gathering as much background information about both of you as possible, including history of sexually transmitted diseases, inherited genetic disorders and your overall state of health.

You may choose to discuss this information with the doctor individually, as many partners prefer to keep sensitive information private, especially when reviewing sexually transmitted diseases. Both of you will have blood tests to assess your risk for HIV, Hepatitis B and C prior to conceiving. In addition, if you suspect you have or may have symptoms of an infection, it is wise to err on the side of caution and have a test for sexually transmitted diseases. Many of the symptoms are discussed on page 22.

Detailed medical history

This is not a test as such, merely a questionnaire that you will complete giving details about your medical and sexual history as well as your current lifestyle – dietary and working patterns; stress levels; smoking, alcohol and drug consumption; current medications taken; illnesses or conditions like epilepsy, anorexia, high blood pressure, depression, etc. and whether there is a family history of genetic disorders. The man will be questioned specifically about problems with libido, ejaculation or erectile function. The woman will be asked about:

- the length of her menstrual cycle
- pains during ovulation
- premenstrual tension
- pain on intercourse
- type of contraception previously used
- any previous miscarriages, stillbirths or children
- known reproductive disorders

Sexual health is an essential part of fertility investigation. Please be honest with your answers even if the information is difficult to talk about. You will benefit in the long run.

Tests for sexually transmitted disease

Because STDs can affect a developing fetus, it is important to ensure that both partners are free of disease. Many STDs are symptomless and can be quietly causing severe damage to the reproductive organs. In the case of chlamydia, about 70 percent of infected women and 50 percent of infected men show no active symptoms. If you have had more than one sexual partner it is advisable that you are tested for any sexually transmitted disease so it can be treated before proceeding. A blood sample or a swab from a potentially affected area will be used depending on the suspected condition.

HIV Human immunodeficiency virus is the virus that causes acquired immune deficiency syndrome (AIDS). AIDS destroys the body's ability to fight infections and the virus is readily passed on to the developing fetus. A blood test can be done to ensure the partners are not carrying the virus prior to conceiving.

Hepatitis B and C cause inflammation of the liver in an infected person. The hepatitis B virus is found in the blood and, to a lesser extent, other bodily fluids such as saliva and semen. It is spread by direct contact with infected fluids during sexual contact or using a needle. Hepatitis C is transmitted by blood-to-blood contact only. A blood test detects the presence of the hepatitis B and C antibodies or parts of the virus itself.

Gonorrhoea, syphilis and chlamydia A swab is taken from the potentially infected area such as the cervix, urethra, penis, anus or throat. A course of antibiotics is usually an effective treatment.

THE WAY GENES WORK

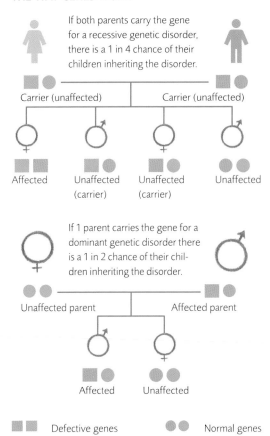

If both parents carry the gene for a recessive genetic disorder, there is a 1 in 4 chance of their children inheriting the disorder.

Carrier (unaffected) — Carrier (unaffected)

Affected | Unaffected (carrier) | Unaffected (carrier) | Unaffected

If 1 parent carries the gene for a dominant genetic disorder there is a 1 in 2 chance of their children inheriting the disorder.

Unaffected parent — Affected parent

Affected | Unaffected

Defective genes   Normal genes

Genetic disorders can be dominant or recessive. Dominant disorders are where anyone who receives a faulty gene from just one parent will have the disorder. An individual will only have a recessive disorder if he or she receives an affected gene from each parent. Achondroplasia (dwarfism) is an example of a dominant genetic disorder, whereas cystic fibrosis is a recessive disorder.

Genetic screening

This is only performed if you have a family history of conditions like sickle cell anaemia, Tay Sachs, or cystic fibrosis. A blood test determines if you have an increased risk of giving birth to a child with a genetic disorder. Often it is not until a couple pair together and review their family histories that it becomes apparent that one or both of them may be carriers of a disorder.

Autoimmune testing

After all the hormonal and structural tests have concluded that there are no known reasons for infertility, autoimmune testing may be carried out. It is estimated that an immune factor may be involved in up to 20 percent of couples with unexplained infertility. To successfully maintain a pregnancy, several immunologic adjustments are required to convert the uterus into a host for the developing embryo and to prevent the fetus and placenta from being rejected. If these mechanisms fail, a woman may experience recurrent miscarriages, infertility or failure to conceive following IVF.

If excessive amounts of antibodies are bound to the sperm they can interfere with sperm motility, affect sperm-egg interaction and reduce the chance of fertilisation. A positive result in a man may be a result of inflammation or injury to the male genitalia. The woman may also be tested for antibodies to sperm cells in her serum that interfere with the sperm mobility and fertilisation.

When to request a test

If the woman has experienced one of the following, it is likely a couple may benefit from immunological screening:

- Two or more miscarriages conceived either naturally or through IVF
- Less than six eggs produced from a stimulated cycle
- One blighted ovum
- Unexplained infertility
- Previous immune problems (rheumatoid arthritis, lupus)
- Previous pregnancies that have shown retarded growth
- One living child and repeat miscarriages while attempting to have a second child

Tests for males

For 32 percent of infertile couples, the male is the one with a problem. Despite their tests being quick and pain free, many men find them extremely unnerving. Sensitivity and understanding is required while the man undergoes investigation.

The primary test is a semen analysis from which significant data is collated to assess the general health of the semen and sperm. Some research suggests that semen should also be screened for antibodies (see page 71). In addition, hormonal and structural problems can be investigated.

Semen analysis

This measures the quantity and quality of the liquid portion of the ejaculate – the semen – and the sperm within the semen.

Sperm count The normal range for sperm is between 40 and 300 million sperm per millilitre of ejaculate. A low sperm count is fewer than 20 million per millilitre of ejaculate. Semen consists of 2 percent sperm and 98 percent fluid. A man typically ejaculates around a teaspoonful (2-6 ml) of fluid. If less semen is ejaculated this may indicate it contains fewer sperm, which would affect fertility. More semen may indicate too much fluid, which would dilute the sperm, also impeding fertility.

Motility (movement) Low sperm motility may reduce the chances of conception, especially when paired with a low sperm count. In a normal semen sample, at least half of the sperm have typical movement. The progression of the sperm is rated on a basis from zero (no motion) to three or higher for sperm that move in a straight line with good speed. If less than half of the sperm are moving, a stain will be used to identify the percentage of dead sperm. This is called a 'sperm viability test'. If over 40 percent of the sperm in the semen analysis are dead, this is called necrospermia. Evidence shows that a man can improve his sperm's motility with conventional and complementary treatments, which are discussed in step 3.

Morphology (shape) A normal sperm has an oval head, a slender midsection and a tail that moves in a wave-like motion. Sperm that have abnormal shapes – large or irregularly shaped heads or defective tails – are often unable to swim effectively or penetrate an egg. The semen analysis evaluates the structure of 200 sperm, and any defects are noted. The more abnormal sperm that are present, the lower the likelihood of fertility.

Common fertility tests

The World Health Organisation provides a definition of a 'normal' sperm count:

- the concentration of sperm should be at least 20 million per ml.

- the total volume of semen should be at least 2ml

- the total number of sperm in the ejaculate should be at least 40 million.

- at least 75 percent of the sperm should be alive (it is normal for up to 25 percent to be dead)

- at least 30 percent of the sperm should be of normal shape and form

- at least 25 percent of the sperm should be swimming with rapid forward movement

- at least 50 percent of the sperm should be swimming forward, even if only sluggishly

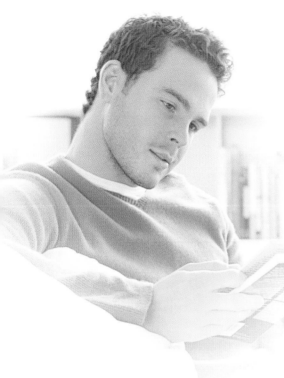

The semen sample is most often collected by masturbation in a private, comfortable room in the fertility centre. In some cases, the sample may be collected at home by masturbation or during intercourse with the use of a special condom that is provided.

Hormone assessment
This blood test can determine the levels of testosterone, follicle-stimulating hormone (FSH), luteinising hormone (LH) and prolactin in the man's body.

Luteinising hormone (LH) is manufactured in the pituitary gland and controls and stimulates the production of testosterone in the testes. Testosterone is responsible for the development of secondary sexual characteristics such as enlargement of the penis, body hair growth and deepening of the voice during puberty. Decreased testosterone levels can occur with physical damage to the testes, excessive alcohol consumption, viral diseases like mumps or genetic diseases, and result in reduced fertility, erectile dysfunction and a decreased sex drive.

Follicle Stimulating hormone (FSH) levels help to determine the reason for a low sperm count. In men, high FSH levels are due to primary testicular failure as a result of developmental defects in testicular growth or to testicular injury through sport.

Further investigations
In some instances the doctor may decide to perform additional tests to ascertain the exact reason behind the infertility. For example, if test results show a reduced testosterone level and a lack of sperm in the semen, a cell culture will identify if it is caused by an infection in the testes. Ultrasound scanning can also detect infection, obstructions and tumours. A testicular biopsy, in which a small sample of tissue is take from one or both testicles and observed under a microscope, may be performed if the sperm count is abnormal and hormone tests are within the normal range. Immunological tests may be performed if both partners have no obvious reason for infertility and are classified as having 'unexplained infertility' (see page 39).

Treatment for male factor infertility both complementary and conventional is discussed in step 3.

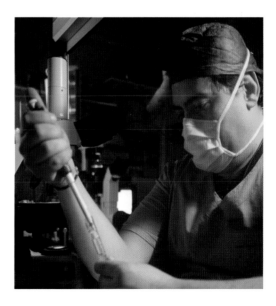

SPERM ASSESSMENT
Should IVF go ahead, sperm will again be extracted from semen prior to the procedure and examined to ensure that only healthy sperm are used.

Tests for females

Due to the complexity of the female reproductive system, there are quite a few tests to perform in order to check all aspects are in full working order.

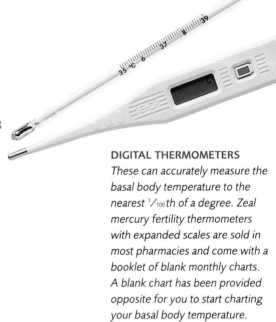

Basal Body Temperature (BBT)

Your basal body temperature is the temperature taken first thing in the morning after several hours of sleep and before any activity, including getting out of bed or talking. Using a special thermometer (see right), it can be measured at home. By taking your temperature every morning you are able to build a monthly profile of the exact day of ovulation and its frequency. Typically the temperature is a little below the recognised normal figure of 37°C (98.6°F). A woman's early morning temperature is lower during the first half of her menstrual cycle by a fraction of a degree. The change in the temperature record from low to high occurs at the time of ovulation. It then shows a drop of 0.1°C to 0.2°C (0.2°F to 0.4°F) at the time of ovulation followed the next day by a rise to the level above that previously recorded.

DIGITAL THERMOMETERS
These can accurately measure the basal body temperature to the nearest $1/100$ th of a degree. Zeal mercury fertility thermometers with expanded scales are sold in most pharmacies and come with a booklet of blank monthly charts. A blank chart has been provided opposite for you to start charting your basal body temperature.

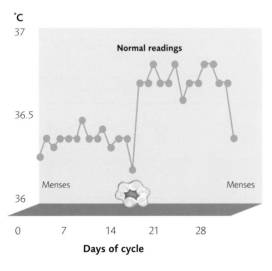

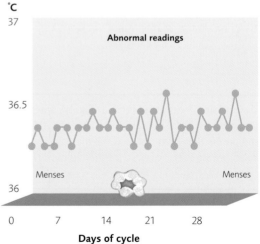

BASAL BODY TEMPERATURE CHARTS
The chart on the left is an example of normal basal body temperature readings over a 28-day menstrual cycle. The chart on the right shows abnormal readings – there is no real discernible rise in basal body temperature over a similar cycle.

Basal Body Temperature Chart

Dates covered: Day ____ Month ____ Year ____ to Day ____ Month ____ Year ____

Cycle Day	1	2	3	4	5	6	7	8	9	10	11	12	13	14	15	16	17	18	19	20	21	22	23	24	25	26	27	28	29	30	31	32	33	34	35	36	37	38	39	40	41	42	43	44	45
Weekday																																													
Date																																													
Time																																													
99.1																																													
99.0																																													
98.9																																													
98.8																																													
98.7																																													
98.6																																													
98.5																																													
98.4																																													
98.3																																													
98.2																																													
98.1																																													
98.0																																													
97.9																																													
97.8																																													
97.7																																													
97.6																																													
97.5																																													
97.4																																													
97.3																																													
97.2																																													
97.1																																													
97.0																																													
96.9																																													

Notes: (List any changes to your routine)

When tests are performed

Most tests are completed at specific times of the menstrual cycle in order to gain an accurate picture of how the body is functioning.

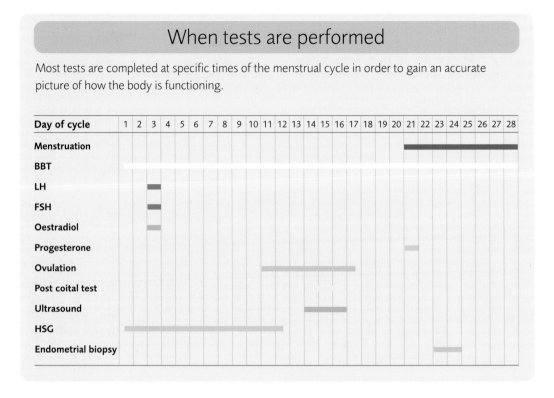

Rhesus (Rh) test

A blood test is done to determine if the blood is Rh-negative or Rh-positive. Eight to 15 percent of pregnant women have Rh-negative blood. This is only a concern if the baby has Rh-positive blood – a possibility if the father is Rh positive. If there is a mismatch, the mother is checked throughout the pregnancy to ensure that her body is not manufacturing antibodies to protect itself from the Rh-positive baby. The Rh incompatability can be prevented by giving the woman an injection of Rh immunoglobulin (anti-D).

Rubella

It is important to check immunity to German measles before getting pregnant. Women without immunity should receive immunisation against rubella provided they avoid pregnancy for a period of three months following immunisation. A blood test determines the occurrence of recent or past infection. Rubella infection in a pregnant woman during the first trimester of pregnancy can result in miscarriage, fetal death or a baby with deafness, mental retardation, heart defects and cataracts.

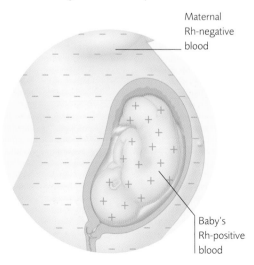

Maternal Rh-negative blood

Baby's Rh-positive blood

RHESUS DISEASE

This occurs when a woman with rhesus-negative blood is pregnant with a rhesus-positive baby. Her body may manufacture antibodies that can attack her baby's red blood cells.

Hormone testing

As part of fertility investigations, a blood test is taken between days 1–3 of the menstrual cycle to determine if the ovaries are functioning normally. To check whether ovulation has occurred, another blood test can be performed on day 21 to check progesterone levels.

Luteinising hormone (LH) When levels of LH (and FSH, see below) peak at mid-cycle they trigger an egg to be released from the ovary – ovulation. This surge of LH also stimulates the ovaries to produce other pregnancy-supporting hormones, particularly oestradiol.

Follicle stimulating hormone (FSH) This hormone stimulates the growth and development of ovarian follicles (eggs) during the follicular phase of the menstrual cycle. A blood test on day three of the menstrual cycle will assess the ovarian reserve and quality of the eggs by measuring FSH levels. Typically, an FSH level under 10 is good, 10 to 15 is borderline and greater than 15 is high.

As women progress towards the age of 40, their ovarian reserve will become depleted as their bodies prepare for peri-menopause. Blood FSH levels do vary from cycle to cycle and you may be asked to perform this test over a three-month period to gain an overall picture of the hormone levels.

If abnormally high or low levels of LH and FSH are present, it is indicative that the body is not functioning normally. For example, about 40 percent of women with polycystic ovarian syndrome will show raised LH levels, which interfere with the development of the egg within the ovarian follicles.

If the reading is borderline or high, your doctor may wish to run additional tests to see what effect the drug clomiphene has on the FSH levels. FSH and oestradiol are measured on day three and then 100 mg of clomiphene medication is taken on days 5 to 9. FSH levels are measured again on day 10. If either day three or day 10 levels are high, this suggests poor ovarian reserve. It also may predict the outcome of fertility treatment. Research has shown that women under 40 with a history of elevated FSH

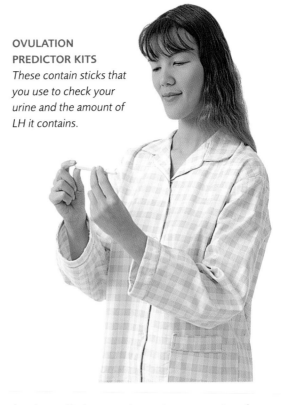

OVULATION
PREDICTOR KITS
These contain sticks that you use to check your urine and the amount of LH it contains.

levels are likely to produce a lower quantity of eggs with IVF but this does not affect their chances of becoming pregnant. However, women over 40 years old tend to have a reduced ovarian response, lower egg yields and lower implantation and pregnancy rates.

Oestradiol (E2) causes the endometrium to thicken for implantation; it naturally decreases with the onset of menopause. Typically a reading between 25-75 pg/ml is normal.

Prolactin is responsible for inducing milk production and stimulating the production of progesterone. Its presence is tested for along with other tests when a woman suffers from irregular periods or the man has a low sex drive.

Progesterone In conjunction with other hormones, progesterone prepares the woman's body for pregnancy. Progesterone levels start to rise when an egg is released from the ovary and continue to rise for several days. If fertilisation does not occur, progesterone levels drop, and menstrual bleeding begins. If levels continue to rise a pregnancy has occurred. A blood test on day 21 indicates whether or not ovulation occurred. Progesterone tests can also assist in the diagnosis of ectopic pregnancies or threatened miscarriages, as in both these situations, progesterone levels do not rise normally as the pregnancy progresses.

Ovulation Tests

Ovulation takes place between days 14 to 16 of the menstrual cycle on average. From day 11 onwards, a sensitive ovulation testing kit can be used, which is available in most pharmacies. Every morning the woman will need to urinate on the testing stick provided. If the LH hormone has been detected, a positive line will appear, indicating ovulation is about to take place. Sexual intercourse in the following two days will maximise the chances of conception.

Post-coital Test

This test measures the sperms' ability to penetrate the cervical mucus and establishes the quality and quantity of cervical mucus.

First the woman uses an ovulation predictor kit to identify the surge in LH that signals ovulation. Then the couple engage in sexual intercourse without the use of lubricants that evening or morning. The woman then visits her doctor or nurse within 4–12 hours of sexual intercourse and a sample by swab is taken from her vagina. The doctor will look at the sample under a microscope to assess the motility of the sperm. The results are given immediately.

Often a second test is required if a poor result is achieved. There are two main reasons for this. The first may be due to 'improper' or late timing; only pre-ovulatory mucus will nourish the sperm and allow them to remain active. The second reason for repeating the test is that as couples have to perform sex on demand, impotence and sexual dysfunction are commonly encountered.

Ultrasound exams

This noninvasive test allows the doctor to view the ovaries, uterus and other internal organs. A probe is placed inside the vagina where it emits ultrasound waves dependent on tissue type, which are then displayed on a monitor.

Throughout the menstrual cycle the thickness of the lining of the uterus changes. Ultrasound can determine when the optimal thickness of 8–10 mm ⅜–½ in) has been achieved. If the lining is thin, it may indicate a hormonal problem.

Ultrasound can also be used to check if the follicle has successfully ruptured at the correct time. Fibroid tumours, abnormalities of the shape of the uterus and the presence of ovarian cysts are also investigated at this time.

Hysterosalpingogram (HSG)

Structural problems, blockages and other disorders of the uterus, the fallopian tubes and the pelvis may be diagnosed through a sophisticated x-ray. A small tube is inserted into the cervix and dye is injected slowly. The flow of the dye into the uterus, out through the fallopian tubes and into the pelvis can be viewed on a screen. This test is performed after a menstrual period and before ovulation. During the injection the woman may feel uterine cramping that may last several hours. After the dye test, there may be a sticky discharge for several hours as the dye is expelled from the uterus. A sanitary napkin is worn instead of a tampon to allow the fluid to escape. Fluid remaining in the pelvic cavity is absorbed by the body without harmful effects. One positive potential side effect of HSG is that

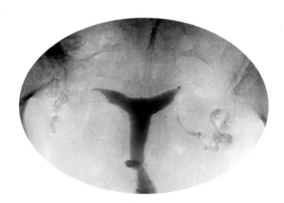

BLOCKED FALLOPIAN TUBES
An HSG has revealed that both fallopian tubes (yellow areas) are blocked by a hydrosalpinx, a fluid-filled swelling of the tube due to pelvic inflammatory disease.

the chance of conception appears to increase
for several cycles after the dye is used.
Because of this, some doctors may prefer to
wait several cycles before proceeding to
the next test, a diagnostic laparoscopy.

Laparoscopy

This procedure is used to view the
outside of the uterus, the ovaries and
the pelvic cavity. The doctor is looking
for scar tissue surrounding the fallopian
tubes, signs of endometriosis and any tubal
disorders. It is performed under general
anaesthetic – usually on an outpatient basis –
and scheduled before ovulation.

A laparascope, or thin telescope, is passed into
the abdomen through an incision near the navel.
A second instrument is inserted through an
incision at the pubic hairline. Carbon dioxide
(CO_2) gas is used to separate the organs inside
the abdominal cavity, making it easier to see the
reproductive organs.

If there are immediate signs of endometriosis
or adhesions, the doctor may choose to
immediately cauterise the tissue to avoid further
unnecessary operations.

Side effects associated with general
anaesthesia include a sore throat, shoulder pain,
a bloated or swollen abdomen and general
stiffness. It is advisable that the woman refrains
from any strenuous activity for a few days. Your
doctor should be able to provide you with
immediate feedback on the state of the pelvic
cavity and any identifiable reasons for infertility.

Hysteroscopy

This procedure allows the doctor to assess if
there are any fibroid tumours, endometrial
polyps, intrauterine scar tissue or other problems
within the uterus.

A narrow telescope-like instrument is inserted
through the vagina and cervix into the cavity of
the uterus. The uterine cavity is then distended
with fluid and visualized. If any defects are
found, they are corrected with operative
hysteroscopy, which involves placing instruments
through ports in the scope that allow doctors to
cut, cauterise, etc., to correct the problem.
The doctor may also take measurements of the

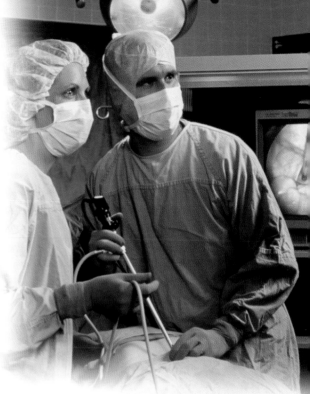

USING A LAPAROSCOPE
*Once you are sedated, a small incision is made in
your abdomen and the thin viewing tube is inserted
allowing your doctor to have a good look inside. CO_2
gas will be pumped in to inflate your abdomen to
make it easier for your doctor to see your organs.*

size and shape of the uterus, which are required
if fertility treatments like IVF are contemplated.
These measurements will help to position the
fertilised embryos to maximise the chances of
implantation. The actual procedure usually takes
two to five minutes. No anaesthesia at all is
needed for most cases of diagnostic hysteroscopy
if a microhysteroscope is used. General
anaesthesia or local anaesthesia can be used if
any operative work is required.

Mild pain and cramping is common after
operative hysteroscopy, but it usually is brief,
lasting perhaps 30 minutes, but possibly up to
eight hours.

Endometrial biopsy

This test involves scraping a small amount of
tissue from the endometrium just before
menstruation in order to assess if a hormone
imbalance exists.

Complementary tests

You and your partner may wish to investigate other reasons why conception has not taken place. Assessing your overall state of health can be done simultaneously with conventional fertility testing or after all the conventional tests have diagnosed you and your partner with 'unexplained infertility'.

Some couples deem unexplained fertility to be the worst diagnosis, as they are unable to move forward to treatment. Others regard this as good news, and decide to focus on improving their health and to keep trying naturally.

Whichever category you fall into, it is important to understand that the body needs certain vitamins and minerals to be in abundance to keep sperm and egg healthy. Sometimes what we perceive to be a good diet may not be supplementing the body in the correct way. Nutritional tests can specifically identify which vitamins and minerals are deficient in your body at any one point in time. It can be heartbreaking to become pregnant after IVF, for example, only to find that you suffer a miscarriage perhaps as a result of having insufficient nutrients to sustain the pregnancy.

Below, I describe the tests available to measure nutritional deficiencies and in the next chapter I will cover which vitamins and minerals are key to conception.

Foresight Programme

A charitable organisation called Foresight has pioneered the importance of a pre-conception diet since 1978. The primary role of the organisation is to promote the importance of good health and nutritional status in both parents before conceiving a baby, and to provide sensible, achievable information and advice on how to do this.

The programme looks at assessing the overall health of both partners before providing a tailored diet and vitamin supplementation plan. Foresight declares that 'it is possible to have uncomplicated pregnancies resulting in strong, healthy and perfectly formed babies, even if the couples previously experienced the distress of miscarriage, stillbirth, birth defects, unexplained infertility, postnatal depression and other health problems.'

Their success lies in the fact that in the modern-day world, our bodies are subjected to numerous pollutants; our lives are hectic and the food we consume is mostly over-processed and over-packaged. Unfortunately, our ability to reproduce is one of the first things to be affected. Many couples experiencing reproductive problems would otherwise consider themselves to be perfectly healthy.

In a study of couples following the Foresight programme, a staggering 89 percent became pregnant and delivered healthy babies simply by following the wholefood diet – a tailored diet and vitamin supplementation programme.

So how can you assess your nutritional status? By using a sample of hair. You remove two tablespoons of hair 2.5 cm (1 in) long from the nape of the neck and send them off for analysis. The Trace Mineral Analysis Laboratory will wash, cook and analyse your hair sample for mineral deficiencies and environmental factors that may be affecting your health (water, detergents, pesticides, lead, etc.).

Within seven days a detailed report is collated comparing your results against the recommended values for each of 19 trace minerals (see example, right). Following the results, a tailored

Foresight

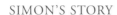

SIMON'S STORY

The source of the lead was not difficult for me to identify, but I knew rectifying the situation would be painful ... emotionally! The cause was my beautiful Lotus Élan – it would have to go, as it was old and still used regular 4-star petrol not unleaded. Happily a satisfactory compromise was reached and a new Elise arrived shortly after! Needless to say the lead levels began to reduce in my body over time! It was a good lesson to both of us about how outside elements may be affecting our health and fertility.

Simon and Marina's hair analysis

	Marina's results	Simon's results	Recommended values mg/kg
Calcium	497	400	400
Magnesium	37.0	42.0	35
Potassium	79.0	81.2	75
Iron	41.0	40.0	30
Chromium	1.89	1.72	0.80
Cobalt	0.19	0.23	0.25
Copper	22.9	21.5	20.0
Manganese	2.09	1.76	1.50
Nickel	1.02	1.42	0.80
Selenium	1.90	1.75	2.25
Zinc	167	173	185
			Threshold values mg/kg
Aluminium	1.95	3.12	2.50
Cadmium	0.34	0.18	0.25
Mercury	0.14	0.17	0.40
Lead	**1.95**	**3.66**	**1.00**
Molybdenum	0.19	0.13	
Vanadium	0.17	0.22	
Rubidium	0.12	0.14	
Sodium	114	93	

supplementation programme is recommended for at least three months prior to conception to enable the body to build up the necessary reserves that may have been deficient. If toxic metals, such as lead, mercury and cadmium are above the threshold levels for successful fetal development, a cleansing programme of vitamins and garlic is recommended until they are within the safe limits. A new hair sample should be taken every three months so that the supplement/cleansing programme can be adjusted until levels are compatible with those ideal for pregnancy. This usually takes four to six months.

Assessing your current nutritional status is key to maximising your chances of conception. A detailed analysis is the only way of truly knowing if your body has the right balance between the essential nutrients and damaging toxins. Foresight contact details are found at the back of the book.

INTERPRETATION:

When Simon and I reviewed our results we were pleased that the majority of essential minerals required were at the recommended levels for conception, some were even in plentiful supply like iron, potassium, magnesium and calcium. However, we became concerned when we realised that both our lead levels were above the threshold values and in Simon's case some 266 percent above what is recommended!

step

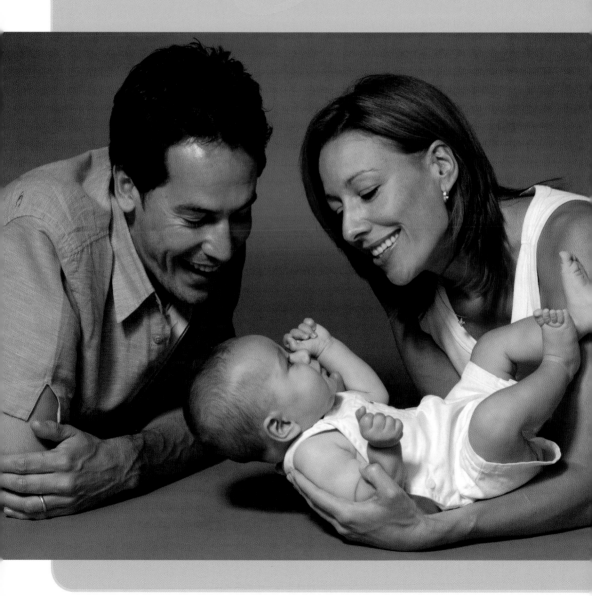

Choose a treatment

for you and your partner

The third and most important step is to find a treatment that will maximise your chances of conception. In today's world, there is a diverse range of fertility treatment available to help couples having problems conceiving. Over the last decade, research has shown that in addition to conventional methods like ovulation induction and IVF, complementary treatments including those based around nutrition, reflexology, herbal medicine, acupuncture and even hypnotherapy can contribute to getting you pregnant. This chapter will look at both the conventional and complementary treatments available and help you confidently select the best way forward.

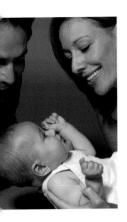

In this chapter, you'll find everything you need to know about the most up-to-date fertility treatments – both conventional and complementary. Before you begin to consider the individual approaches described below, you might like to refer to the chart on the opposite page. I've designed this to help you find out whether you should see a professional right away or whether there are things you can do on your own to improve your fertility – like making some changes to your diet or giving up smoking, for example. However, one of the most important considerations as to when to seek professional help is your age. The older you are, the less likely you will conceive and be able to carry a baby to term.

The effect of age

Before you look in detail at the treatments, it is important that I re-emphasise the importance of your age in choosing an approach. While it is important that you change an unsupportive lifestyle, improve your diet, and reduce unhealthy influences like stress in your life, it would be foolish to suggest that if you are actively having sex and are over 35 you wait a whole year before visiting your doctor to commence testing. This may contravene advice from some health professionals but, realistically, age plays a vital role in a woman's ability to become pregnant and carry a pregnancy to term. By waiting you are simply adding to your problems. My recommendation is to simultaneously change your lifestyle and diet while undergoing fertility investigations.

With advancing age, many biological changes take place which work against conceiving and carrying the pregnancy to term; many of these have been discussed earlier. From age 30 to 35, there is a gradual decline in the ability of women to become pregnant; after age 40, there is a sharp decline. Also, the chance of miscarriage and chromosomal abnormalities, such as those that cause Down's syndrome, increase with age. Even the success of in vitro fertilisation and other similar procedures decreases with advancing age.

The table on page 85 outlines the various treatment options. It shows who can benefit, what type of treatment it is and how much time

Age and fertility

The results of a study looking at the reproductive span and rate of conception among Hutterite women showed the following:

by age 30, 7% of couples were infertile

by age 35, 11% of couples were infertile

by age 40, 33% of couples were infertile

at age 45, 87% of couples were infertile

and money is involved. In addition, each treatment is rated on a scale of 1–5 (1 being the least) as to how invasive it is. Many couples prefer to try a gentle approach prior to opting for the more invasive ones. By invasive, I mean methods that require internal scans, blood tests and potentially internal investigations. Many treatments are successful without this type of intervention.

TREATMENTS OVERVIEW
The table on the right aims to give you an overview on the key aspects of each treatment type to help you choose the right path for your treatment.

WHAT'S YOUR PATH TO PREGNANCY?

Less than 35 years old   **Greater than 35 years old**

Just started trying for a baby   Actively having sex for more than 1 year   Trying for a few months (3–6)

▼

Improve diet/take supplements ◄········

▼

Exercise

▼

Change lifestyle (give up alcohol, smoking etc.)

▼

Use relaxation techniques/reduce stress

▼

Learn more about ideal time for conception, use Billings method/ovulation kits

▼

After 1 year of trying

···► **See doctor for testing**

▼

Identify infertility reason

▼

Unexplained infertility?
Male infertility?
Hormonal problems?
Structural problems?

▼

Choose a treatment
Diet and nutrition
Ovulation tracking
Reflexology
Acupuncture
Herbal medicine
Hypnotherapy
Ovulation induction
IVF
Egg/sperm donation

Treatment	Male/ Female	Complementary or conventional	Time required	Cost (£)	Gentle Invasive (1–5)
Diet and nutrition	Both	Complementary	>3 months	0	1
Ovulation tracking	Female	Complementary	6wks–3months	0	1
Reflexology	Female	Complementary	>3 months	£	2
Acupuncture	Both	Complementary	>3 months	£	2
Herbal medicine	Both	Complementary	>3 months	£	1
Hypnotherapy	Female	Complementary	6wks–3months	££	2
Ovulation induction	Female	Conventional	6wks–3months	££	4
IVF (in-vitro fertilisation)	Both	Conventional	4–6 weeks	££££	5
Egg /sperm donation	Both	Conventional	4–6 weeks	££££	5

Complementary treatments

Complementary treatments tend to be less invasive and costly than conventional fertility treatments. In this section we will review the treatments and discuss how they can specifically improve your chance of getting pregnant.

Diet and nutrition

You may already be a firm believer in the benefits of maintaining a healthy diet or you may be sceptical as to how the food you eat can help your fertility. Either way, there is enough evidence to suggest that your diet may need tweaking to prepare yourself for pregnancy and carry a baby to full term. Sperm and egg production, fertilisation, implantation and growing a baby for nine months all require an abundance of essential nutrients. Unfortunately, despite your efforts to eat healthily, the food you eat is unlikely to contain all that you need, which is why we advocate a vitamin and mineral supplementation plan. Let's look at what the ideal pre-conception diet should consist of and where you can get your essential nutrients.

Why is nutrition a treatment for infertility?
Couples who have had problems conceiving have become pregnant by changing their diet and lifestyle. A three-year study of 367 infertile couples showed that after making the necessary dietary changes, 86 percent became pregnant naturally (see page 40). The Foresight Organisation confidently demonstrates the benefits of changing your diet and nutrition and throughout this section I will provide you with an overview of their recommendations.

Unexplained causes currently account for 20 percent of infertility cases. In these cases, tests have shown there are no problems with hormones, the structure of the reproductive organs or sperm, yet after actively trying for over a year, pregnancy has not occurred. In these cases, diet and nutrition may be able to assist couples in conceiving. Despite efforts to live a healthy lifestyle, it is becoming more difficult to consume all the essential nutrients required for

conception; today's foods are over processed and covered with harmful chemicals such as pesticides. The foods that you eat and drink affect your health and can cause infertility. It is amazing to think that couples have conceived by changing their diet alone, but it is true.

Even if a cause for your infertility has been diagnosed as requiring conventional treatment, research has shown that a healthy diet will reduce the risk of a miscarriage and assist you in carrying a baby to full term. Miscarriage can occur due to a bad diet, lack of essential vitamins or a harmful lifestyle.

Complementary treatments work well on their own as well as in conjunction with conventional treatments. Of all the complementary treatments, diet and nutrition is the one I recommend you implement immediately, as the benefits to you and a potential baby are so significant. Another added benefit is that it costs very little to make the changes outlined in this section. Although I require IVF to have a baby – both my fallopian tubes having been removed – I also follow a pre-conception diet, cut out harmful toxins and use complementary treatments like reflexology to help me relax while undergoing IVF. I feel happy in the knowledge that I am doing everything I can to maximise my chances of conceiving and preventing a miscarriage.

Following a diet and nutrition programme does require dedication and determination; however, if you are already reading this book, you are dedicated and determined to maximise your chances of conception, so it should be easy!

How do you establish if your body has the right balance of nutrients? If you have already had a vitamin and mineral assessment (see page 80), you will be aware of what key nutrients are lacking in your diet and will hopefully have started taking the essential supplements to boost your fertility. If you have decided not to have a hair mineral analysis, you are still able to evaluate your current diet and make the necessary changes by reviewing your diet against the 'good' and 'bad' foods covered in this section. Remember the earlier you start making the changes, the sooner you may become pregnant! Typically it takes three months for you and your partner's body to realise the benefits of dietary changes.

What is a healthy diet? For our purposes of increasing your chances of conception it is a diet that provides your body with all the necessary nutrients to conceive and carry a healthy baby to full term while eliminating all the harmful toxic chemicals that interfere with this process. Most of the toxic chemicals have been discussed in step 1 (see page 50), but to refresh your memory, the most damaging to you and your baby-making chances are caffeine, cigarettes, alcohol, recreational drugs, lead, mercury, pesticides and herbicides.

The pre-conception diet

There has been an enormous amount of research in the field of nutrition for conception and pregnancy. The Foresight programme has amalgamated all the findings from eminent scientists in the field to create a wholefood diet approach. The old adage of 'you are what you eat' is even more important when creating a baby as you are laying down the foundations for your future offspring's growth and development. Bear in mind that when I refer to 'diet', I do not mean a weight-loss or 'fad' diet. Instead, it is a plan designed to increase the essential nutrients for conception and pregnancy.

The pre-conception diet focuses on eating the right foods in abundance. On page 45, I discussed the importance of being the right weight for pregnancy and how being under- or overweight affects your fertility. Some guidelines were outlined to help you achieve the right BMI (body mass index) prior to trying for a baby. I don't recommend you start dieting while trying for a baby; achieve the right weight first, then concentrate on building the necessary reserves for pregnancy with the pre-conception diet.

Eat organic

The majority of foods you consume should be organic. All supermarkets now have an extensive range of organic products. Eating organic food is very important in the pre-conception diet as it is free of the harmful herbicides and pesticides that can affect fertility. If you can't go all-organic, shop at supermarkets that ban controversial pesticides and try to source food locally to ensure maximum freshness and a smaller chance of it having been sprayed with post-harvest pesticides and waxes for safe travelling.

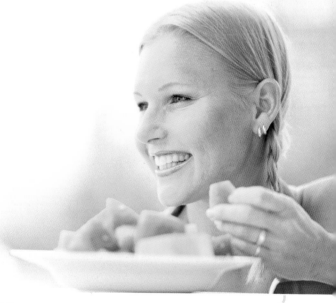

A good pre-conception diet consists of carbohydrates, proteins, fats, fibre and plenty of clean water. Within these groups are found the various vitamins and minerals essential for your well-being and pregnancy.

Carbohydrates

These supply your body with its primary source of energy – glucose. Glucose is a type of sugar and is the main source of fuel for your muscles, nervous system and brain. There are two main types, simple carbohydrates (sugars) and complex carbohydrates (starches and fibres). Both are healthy. Simple carbohydrates occur naturally in fruit, vegetables, milk and honey. In this form they contain nutrients. However, when simple sugars are processed in the form of cakes, biscuits, sweets and fizzy drinks, they are stripped of any minerals and vitamins, and the pure sugar provides a 'quick fix' when it enters the bloodstream, disturbing blood sugar levels.

These 'empty calories' are unhealthy and do not provide any nutrients needed for conception and pregnancy. On the other hand, complex carbohydrates, which also contain naturally occurring sugars, are digested easily and release energy in a slow balanced way essential for body functioning. Complex carbohydrates are found in grains and starchy vegetables such as potatoes and sweetcorn.

Proteins

These are responsible for building and repairing enzymes, muscles, organs, tissues and hair and are often referred to as the body's 'building blocks'. Proteins are made of amino acids, which are broken down in the body to form other amino acids. The role amino acids have in maintaining our health and fertility is only now becoming understood. Two amino acids, spermadine and aspermine play a major role in the synthesis of semen. Men with low sperm

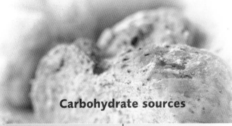

Carbohydrate sources

Good	Bad
Wholegrains, oats, wholemeal pasta, rye, maize, millet	Sugar
	White flour
	White bread
Wholemeal bread	White pasta
Oatmeal	Sweets/biscuits/puddings
Brown rice	
Buckwheat	Coloured carbonated drinks
Fresh vegetables (raw, steamed)	Jams/jellies
Fruit	Undiluted fruit juice
Potatoes	
Honey	
Beans and pulses (kidney beans, chick peas, lentils)	

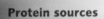

Protein sources

Good	Bad
Organic meat	Bought pies
Organic poultry	TV dinners, microwave dinners
Organic fish	
Organic milk	Sausages/hamburgers/hotdogs
Organic cheese	
Organic nuts, pulses and seeds	Salamis
	Paté and processed meats

counts also have low levels of spermadine and aspermine. Fortunately, with the right foods and supplements, it is possible to raise the levels and help to improve sperm count.

Fats

These provide energy, help build cell walls and balance hormones. 'Fat' is a generic term that encompasses both good and bad fats. Many fats are vital to our health and fertility and should be consumed as part of the pre-conception diet; others are to be avoided.

Saturated fats, which are usually solid at room temperature, are harmful to your body and cause high blood cholesterol, hardening of the arteries and heart disease. Red meat, lamb, pork, lard, butter, cream, milk and other dairy products made from whole milk all contain saturated fats. Fat which has undergone a chemical process called hydrogenation (common in margarine and shortening), should also be limited in your diet.

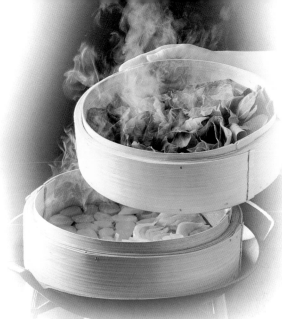

Fat sources

Good	Bad
Extra virgin olive oil, sesame oil, sunflower oil, peanut oil	Red meat, lamb, pork
	Full-fat dairy milk, cream
Avocado	Butter
Peanut butter	Palm oil/palm kernel oil
Unhydrogenated margarine	Margarine
	Low fat spread
Fish oils, linseed and flax oil	Pastries/pies/biscuits
	Potato crisps
Mackerel, sardines	Chocolate
Nuts and seeds (safflower, sesame and sunflower, pumpkin)	Sweets
	Ice cream
Corn and soy beans	Cereal bars
Sea vegetables	Fried food
Sweet potatoes	
Walnuts	

Unsaturated fats, which are usually liquid at room temperature, are 'good' fats and are essential for functioning of the brain, nervous system, immune and reproductive systems. These fats are found in oils, fish, nuts and seeds and they contain Essential Fatty Acids (EFAs). The body is unable to make them so it is essential you eat EFAs. Omega-3, omega-6 and omega-9 can be bought as an oil supplement which can be added to your daily food such as salad.

Food preparation

For a healthy diet to be optimised, fruit should be eaten fresh and vegetables should be raw or lightly steamed. Poultry and fish should be baked, grilled or steamed. By doing so, you are ensuring that most of the essential vitamins and minerals are not lost during the cooking process.

Fibre

Found in fruit and vegetables, nuts, seeds, pulses and whole grains, fibre is essential for maintaining a healthy digestive system and eliminating toxic matter from the body. Several causes of infertility like PCOS (polycystic ovarian syndrome), endometriosis and fibroids are thought to be associated with excess oestrogen levels in the body. Fibre helps to reduce or alleviate the symptoms associated with these illnesses by preventing oestrogen from being reabsorbed back into the blood. Vegetarian women tend to excrete three times more old oestrogen than meat-eating women. This explains why the diet most highly recommended for women with these conditions is a high-fibre, low-fat one, which is mainly vegetarian.

Water

Essential to our health, water forms over 60 percent of our body weight and is involved in every chemical reaction. In today's world it is very important to ensure we drink water that is of good quality and free from pollutants. If you are concerned about the quality of your tap water, you can contact your local water supplier and request a summary of the toxicity report. Always use filtered or bottled water to ensure that harmful nitrates, lead and toxins have been eliminated and the useful trace elements required are present. The recommended daily amount to ensure your body is working at its optimum is eight glasses of water a day.

Vitamins and Minerals

It is widely accepted that certain vitamins and minerals are vital before, during and after pregnancy. You only have to visit your local doctor's surgery to see the numerous posters about the importance of taking folic acid supplements to help prevent neural tube defects like spina bifida. There are several other vitamin and minerals essential to your reproductive health, and which can make a difference to your fertility. In the chart, you will see how each vitamin and mineral can help to maximise your chance of conception, maintain pregnancy, and what the consequence may be if you are deficient. Please bear in mind that some of the conditions are a result of serious deficiencies and one would hope that with a healthy balanced diet most will be avoided.

Summary

In summary, the pre-conception diet means that you cut out white flour products, sugar, processed foods, red meat and unhealthy snacks like crisps and eat a diet abundant in organic fruit, vegetables, fish, nuts, seeds and whole grain products; drink at least eight glasses of purified water a day and supplement your diet with the recommended vitamins and minerals. By doing so, you will be maximising your chances of conception!

Fat Soluble Vitamins

The body can accumulate stores against shortages, however to conceive and maintain a pregnancy the stores may need supplementing.

Required for	If deficient
Vitamin A 600 mcg/day RNI*	
Production of male and female sex hormones, helps to regulate thyroid gland. Take in moderation, an excess can cause birth defects.	A fetus may have eye defects, cleft palate, cleft lip, undescended testicles, neural tube defects. A baby may be stillborn.
Vitamin E 15–30 iu RNI*	
Muscle strength and hormone production. Helps with metabolising essential fatty acids and selenium, sperm function. May help prevent miscarriage and ease labour by strengthening the muscles.	Babies may be anaemic or jaundiced; have weak muscles, retarded heart development, brain, lung and kidney damage, backward development and squint.
Vitamin K 45–80 mcg RNI*	
Blood clotting; it is given to some women at the time of birth and to newborn babies to reduce the risk of internal bleeding and haemorrhages. Helps to reduce excessive menstrual flow.	Can increase the tendency to haemorrage in the mother and baby.
Essential fatty acids (Omega-3,6,9) 700–1000 mg/day RNI*	
Production of sex and adrenal hormones, important in regulating hormones. Essential for fetal brain development.	Linked to pre-eclampsia.

*RNI recommended nutrient intake

Essential vitamins for reproductive health

Water Soluble Vitamins

These vitamins are readily absorbed in water and are lost when passing urine.

Required For	If deficient
Folic acid 400 mcg RNI*	
Growth and division of body and red blood cells. Aids in transmission of genetic code. Essential for metabolising zinc.	Neural tube defects like spina bifida. Neural tube development takes place between days 26–27 of the embryo's life which is why taking folic acid before pregnancy is essential to build up reserves.
Vitamin B$_1$ (Thiamin) 0.8 mcg/day RNI*	
Release of energy from food, digestion, nervous system and help with dealing with stress.	In pregnancy it can lead indirectly to a loss of appetite, nausea and tiredness, which can result in low birth weight. Depression may also occur.
Vitamin B$_2$ (Riboflavin) 1.1 mcg/day RNI*	
Healthy eyes, mouth, skin, nails and hair.	Cleft palate and short limbs. Increased risk of miscarriage and low birth weight.
Vitamin B$_5$ (Pantothenic acid) 5–10 mcg/day RNI*	
Involved in the body's immune system and is needed to release energy from fats, carbohydrates and protein.	In animals, fetal abnormalities including cleft palate, heart defects and club foot and miscarriage has been noted. Similar problems are suspected in humans.
Vitamin B$_6$ 1.6–2.2 mcg/day RNI*	
Reproductive health, formation of female sex hormones and important in regulating oestrogen and progesterone levels. Some nutritionists recommend taking up to 50 mg/day.	Premenstrual tension, nausea and vomiting. Babies born with B6 deficiency have abnormalities including cleft palate.
Vitamin C 60 mcg RNI*	
Provides resistance to infections, poison, toxins such as lead, helps healing and absorption of iron. May increase this to 500 mcg/day when trying to conceive.	Causes sperm to clump together and reduces fertility.

Minerals

Required For	If deficient
Zinc 30 mcg RNI*	
Health and maintenance of hormone levels in men and women. Important component of semen. Helps cell division of fertilised egg.	Low levels result in low sperm count and motility leading to infertility. Low birth weight of baby.
Selenium 100 mcg RNI*	
Fighting infections, combines with toxins to eliminate them from the body, helps against chromosome problems.	In USA 25% of babies who die each year are found to be deficient in selenium and/or Vitamin E.
Calcium 800–1200 mcg RNI*	
Strong teeth and bones, nerve and muscle function. Vital for the growth of the fetus and health of the mother.	Low levels associated with low birth weight and premature babies.
Copper No RNI*	
Aids development of brain, bones, nerves and connective tissue.	Deficiency is rare, copper excess can be toxic.
Iron 10–18 mcg RNI*	
Red blood cell production, resistance to infections, helps to prevent miscarriage.	Anaemia. In babies, eye defects, slow growth, bone and brain defects.
Magnesium 270–350 mcg RNI*	
Health of circulatory system, nerves and muscles.	May be associated with miscarriage and premature birth, low-birth-weight babies.
Manganese 1.4 mg/day RNI*	
Skeletal development, improves memory, nerve function.	Babies with congenital malformations have significantly lower levels of manganese than babies without malformations.
Potassium No RNI*	
Controlling activity of heart muscles, nervous system and kidneys.	Linked to poor sperm motility. In the embryo, abnormalities of the kidneys may occur.

Sources of vitamins and minerals

This table highlights the foods that contain the essential vitamins and minerals necessary for reproductive health.

Folic Acid

Brewer's yeast
Whole grains
Green vegetables
Wheatgerm
Milk
Root vegetables
Oysters
Salmon
Dates
Mushrooms
Orange juice
Alfalfa sprouts
Chickpeas

EFAs

Unrefined oils
(cold pressed)
Nuts
Nut butters (cold
pressed)
Green leafy
vegetables
Seeds
Fatty fish

Vitamin A

Milk
Butter
Cheese
Yoghurt
Egg yolk
Fatty fish
Fish liver oil
Parsley
Kale
Spinach
Greens
Chard
Carrots
Red peppers

Vitamin E

Unrefined oils
(cold pressed)
Whole grains
Wheatgerm
Milk
Egg yolk
Green leafy
vegetables
Lettuce
Avocado
Peanuts
Pumpkin &
sesame seeds
Nut butter (cold
pressed)
Soya beans

Vitamin B$_1$ (Thiamine)

Whole grains
Hazelnuts
Dried beans
Peas
Lentils
Soya beans
Peanut butter
Brewer's yeast
Wheatgerm
Pork
Ham
Eggs
Green leafy
vegetables
Fresh pineapple

Vitamin B$_2$ (Riboflavin)

Brewer's Yeast
Wheatgerm
Whole grains
Green vegetables
Milk
Yoghurt
Eggs
Soya Beans
Peas
Butter
Cheese
Mushrooms

Vitamin B$_6$ (Pyridoxine)

Brewer's yeast
Whole grains
Molasses
Wheatgerm
Peanuts
Mushrooms
Potatoes
Yeast extract
Oatflakes
Soya beans
Seaweeds
Sunflower seeds
Salmon
Beef
Mackerel

Pantothenic Acid (Vitamin B$_5$)

Brewer's yeast
Whole grains
Wheatgerm
Yeast
Mushrooms
Green vegetables
Beans
Chickpeas
Soya beans
Brown rice
Avocado

Vitamin B$_{12}$ (Cobalamin)

Milk
Eggs
Cheese
Seaweeds
Oysters
Beef
Pork
Sardines
Tuna
Turkey
Chicken

" KAREN'S STORY – A CASE OF
LEAD IN THE WATER?

We had been trying for a baby for over four years. Hair analysis revealed a towering lead level in both of us. I had a very high copper level and low levels of zinc, manganese and other essential minerals. I am a lacto-vegetarian (which can mean less zinc in the diet) and many years before had been using the contraceptive pill. Our toxic chemicals were so high that programmes of cleansing and supplementing went on for over a year, but our patience was finally rewarded. Our little boy was born, weighing 6lb 14 oz. Recently, thinking about having another child, we sent hair for analysis again. This was wise, as my husband's lead had crept back significantly. At work he drinks tea made with unfiltered water.

Iron

Lean meats
Apricots
Eggs
Whole grains
Molasses
Eggs
Shellfish
Dried fruits
Seaweeds
Sunflower seeds
Dried fruits
Watermelon
Mushrooms
Beetroot

Zinc

Shellfish
Whole grains
Brewer's yeast
Wheatgerm
All fruit
All vegetables
Bananas
Seeds
Seaweeds
Ginger root
Nuts
Egg yolk
Oysters
Meat
Fish
Poultry

Vitamin C

All citrus fruits
Apples
Apricots
Bananas
Blackcurrants
Clementines
Grapefruits
Grapes
Guavas
Limes
Mangos
Melons
Nectarines

Selenium

Brewer's yeast
Whole grains
Garlic
Eggs
Fish and shellfish
Wholemeal bread
Cheddar cheese
Carrots
Turnip
Mushroom

Copper

Whole grains
Green vegetables
Shellfish
Crab
Wholemeal bread
Lentils
Olives
Nuts
Raisins

Calcium

Milk
Cheese
Bone broth
Green vegetables
Egg yolk
Shellfish
Salmon
Prunes
Almonds
Nuts
Seeds
Oranges
Papayas
Watermelon

Manganese

Whole grains
Wheatgerm
Seeds
Leafy vegetables
Brewer's yeast
Egg
Onions
Green beans
Parsley
Strawberries
Bananas
Apples
Pineapple
Cherries

Potassium

Watercress
Bananas
Avocado
Elderberries
Papayas
Dried apricots
Nuts
Red peppers
All fresh fruit
All vegetables

Magnesium

Nuts – cashews
Milk
Eggs
Green vegetables
Seafoods
Whole grains
Sprouted seed
and grains
Seafood
Avocado
Dates
Dried apricots
Brown rice
Bananas

Diet for sufferers of PCOS, endometriosis and fibroids

Some women reading this book may already know the reason for their infertility and be looking for ways to increase their chance of getting pregnant. If you have PCOS, endometriosis or fibroids it has been proved that a change in diet can significantly reduce your symptoms and increase your fertility. It is thought these conditions are a result of too much oestrogen circulating in the body. Switch from a high-fat high-protein diet to a low-fat high-fibre diet. Eating lots of fibre helps to maintain a healthy blood sugar level and prevents oestrogen from being reabsorbed back into the body.

The recommendations follow the same principles as the pre-conception diet outlined above with additional requirements specific to these conditions. The details of the foods to avoid and vitamins and herbs to take can be found on page 26. Follow the pre-conception diet and specific recommendations for at least three months and monitor your symptoms. You should begin to feel a difference during this time!

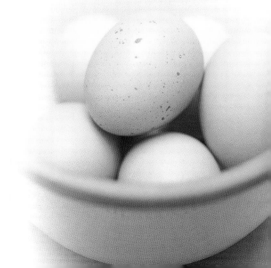

The three-month plan

A special pre-conception plan has been created to help you make the necessary changes to your diet and lifestyle while starting the process of fertility investigations. While gaining optimum health for conception, I think it is important to simultaneously visit your doctor to start the ball rolling with the basic fertility investigations, e.g. screening for infections. Some of you may already know the reason for your infertility and do not need to have any further investigations. If so, you are able to start the three-month plan straightaway in the knowledge that each week you are gaining better reproductive health and maximising your chances of conception. A three-month period is deemed sufficient amount of time to rid your body of unwanted toxins, change your diet and to begin to feel the benefits of your hard work. You will feel less tired and lethargic and feel positive and energised knowing you are doing all you can to maximise your chances of conception.

MONTH 1

This is the hardest part of your three-month programme. You need to set a date for you and your partner to start and make these important changes to your diet and lifestyle. You will both need to be fully committed and supportive of each other as you embark on these changes. Choose a week to start when your social diary is quiet and work pressures are at a minimum – this will make it easier to complete the transition.

WEEK 1

Recommended changes this week are:
- Give up caffeine, smoking, alcohol and recreational drugs;
- Start a 3-day detoxification programme.

Give it up!

Easier said than done, I should know! If any of your friends and family know you are trying for a baby and observe that you are still smoking and drinking, they may be nagging you and rightly so. Having been a social smoker and drinker, I know that when you are under the strain of

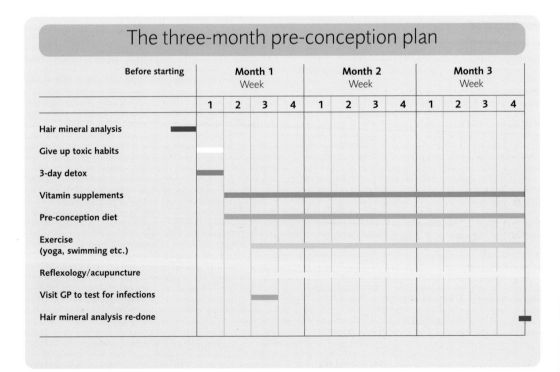

The three-month pre-conception plan

	Before starting	Month 1 Week				Month 2 Week				Month 3 Week			
		1	2	3	4	1	2	3	4	1	2	3	4
Hair mineral analysis	▬												
Give up toxic habits													
3-day detox													
Vitamin supplements													
Pre-conception diet													
Exercise (yoga, swimming etc.)													
Reflexology/acupuncture													
Visit GP to test for infections													
Hair mineral analysis re-done													

trying for a baby it can be stressful, and smoking a cigarette and drinking a glass of wine can do a lot to make you relax. That said, smoking and drinking also worsen the situation by reducing your chances of conception. I had a serious chat with myself one day and decided to muster up all my motivation to stop otherwise I would remain in this vicious circle. If I was serious about having a baby, I had to stop there and then! I immediately did a detox and once I saw the results, there was no going back!

Do whatever works for you to give up; I am no expert in helping people give up, I just know that you will significantly increase your chances of getting pregnant when you do. If you need to seek help, do so, or find another way to relieve stress; take up exercise or go for a weekly massage or avoid all the associations you may have with smoking and drinking. It may be difficult for some of you but it is definitely worth it in the long run, especially if you can visualise yourself with a little baby in your arms!

If you do not smoke, drink or take recreational drugs, you are well on your way to optimum reproductive health. I still recommend you perform a three-day detox as, unknown to you, other toxins like pesticides, mercury and lead may be prevalent in your system. Ideally, the aim is to start the pre-conception diet with a clean healthy body and subsequently to build up the essential vitamins and minerals necessary for conceiving a healthy baby.

What is a detox?

Detoxification is the process of eliminating toxins from the body, which have accumulated as a consequence of stress, poor dietary habits, pollution, cigarettes, drugs and alcohol. In the last five years there has been an enormous amount of focus on 'detox' diets in magazines and several books now exist on the subject. Understanding which detoxification programme is ideal for you can be difficult as they range in length and severity. For example, you can do a one-day, three-day, seven-day or even a 28-day detox. You can buy ready-made over-the-counter herbal 'detox' packs or juice fruits. 'Die hard' detoxers complete a water fast or a liver flush.

Over the years, Simon and I have tried most of them with varying degrees of success. I even went on a 10-day juice fast following IVF treatment to rid my body of the fertility drugs, which made me feel so unwell. The plan we find the easiest to incorporate into our daily lives and work patterns is a three-day juice detox. The main benefit is the speed at which toxins are eliminated from the body; the results are almost immediate and it seems a lot can be achieved in a short period of time compared to other programmes. Longer detoxes are gentler and can take weeks for the benefits to be realised. For Simon and I it is easy to take three days out of our busy lives to focus solely on this task –– typically starting on a Friday morning and by Sunday night the benefits are apparent, leaving us ready to start the pre-conception diet on Monday. However if you feel happier completing another type of detox, please do! The most important factor is that your body is cleansed of harmful toxins prior to starting the diet.

What are the benefits of detoxing?

Detoxing claims to encourage the body's natural self-cleansing mechanisms and gives the digestive system a much-needed rest. Body organs like the kidneys, the skin, the liver, the

What do I need?

For this three-day detox you will need:

- Dry skin brush

- Juicer

- Lots and lots of organic raw fruit and vegetables like apples, pears, carrots, bananas, greens, spinach and celery

- Psyllium husk powder (available at pharmacies and health food shops)

- Bentonite (available at pharmacies and health food shops)

- Herbal teas (e.g. nettle, camomile, lemon and ginger)

lungs and the lymphatic system all benefit from the removal of unwanted toxins. The benefits are more energy, clearer skin, improved sleep, greater mental clarity and a more efficient immune system.

If at any time you are concerned about the detox or your health, seek advice from a medical practitioner or nutritionist before starting.

How will I feel?

This depends on how toxic your body is. If you and your partner drink tea and coffee, smoke every day, drink a bottle of wine each night and eat TV dinners, you may feel absolutely terrible by day three when all the toxins are circulating in your bloodstream having been purged from the cells, tissues and muscles of your body. Headaches, tiredness, lethargy, feeling cranky and emotional are common symptoms. It is essential to drink plenty of water – two litres a day to help to eliminate the toxins from your body. On the following days (usually five to

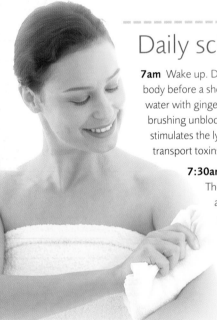

Daily schedule for the 3-day detox

7am Wake up. Dry skin brush the whole body before a shower. Drink warm hot water with ginger or lemon. Dry skin brushing unblocks the pores and stimulates the lymphatic system to transport toxins to the liver and kidney.

7:30am Colon sweep shake. The volcanic bentonite attracts the toxins and the psyllium husk powder binds it to aid removal from the body.

10am Detox juice.

11:30am Colon shake.

1:30pm Detox juice.

2–6pm Spend this time relaxing: reading, walking, doing yoga, swimming.

3pm Colon shake.

6:30pm Dinner – hot potassium vegetable broth.

9:30pm Take enema. Enema kits can be bought from most pharmacies. This will help your body eliminate the daily toxic matter that has accumulated in your bowels. If you are not happy to do this, then just gently massage your stomach and lower abdomen each night.

Colon Sweep Shake

Put 2 teaspoons of volcanic bentonite in 150 ml of water. Shake well in an air-tight container until the lumps have dissolved. Add 2 teaspoons of psyllium husk powder. Top up with apple juice until 500 ml. Shake well, pour into glass, and drink immediately.

Detox Juice

Use juicer to make a large pitcher (about 2 pints) of juice. Choose from one of the following options. Apples and pears or apples and carrots or carrot and orange.

Hot Potassium Vegetable Broth

Each night make this broth fresh. Add potatoes, greens, celery, kelp (if available) and green vegetables to a large pan of boiling water. Bring to the boil, simmer for at least half an hour. Purée in a blender then add hot filtered water until it is a watery broth. ENJOY as much as possible. Add raw grated garlic, ginger or lemon to enhance the taste.

Drink herbal tea any time (you can also boil raw ginger and mix with organic honey or lemon). Throughout the day drink at least one-and-a-half litres of water in addition to the juice and herbal teas to help flush out the toxins. Try to get at least eight hours' sleep. Listen to your body; if you have a headache or are feeling unwell, lie down to give your body a chance to complete the cleansing process.

seven), you will feel much better. Your eyes will sparkle, your skin will glow and you will feel totally energised. Having been through the detox and seen the outcome, you will hopefully be averse to ingesting any more toxins and falling into your old habits. On day four, aim to start the pre-conception diet and maintain this eating plan for up to three months until you have had another hair mineral analysis done or conceived a baby.

At the end of day 3, start preparing yourself for the beginning of the pre-conception diet. The first day after the detox, eat light, easily digestible foods like salads and fish as this avoids putting too much strain on the digestive system straightaway. Avoid dairy and wheat products for a couple of days. You may still be feeling sluggish, which can indicate that your body is quite toxic and it may take a few more days of very light eating to complete the process. The good news is, you are cleansing your body; the toxins are coming out!

OPTIONAL – At the end of the 3-day detox, you may see additional benefits if you have colonic irrigation. Again seek medical advice from a nutritionist or GP if you have not done this before or are concerned about your health.

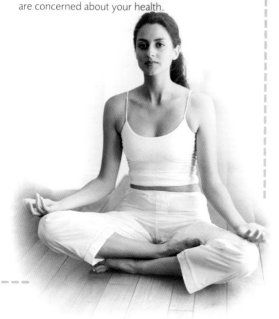

Good food choices

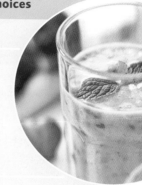

Breakfast

Muesli and fruit, oat porridge, fruit smoothies, yoghurt and fruit, boiled egg on wholemeal toast, organic orange juice, herbal tea (camomile, dandelion, nettle).

Morning Snack

Dried apricots, banana, cheese on ryvita, grapes, celery and carrot sticks with hummus, smoothies, any fruit, nuts and seeds, rye toast.

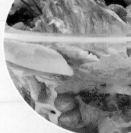

Lunch

Any salad full of raw vegetables sprinkled with seeds with or without organic fish (tuna) and chicken, vegetable soups with rye bread, grilled sardines and salad, grilled goats' cheese with fresh raspberry sauce, fruit, yoghurt.

Afternoon Snack

Banana, raisins, apple, herbal tea..

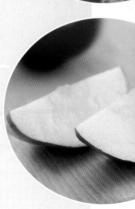

Dinner

Fresh organic fish or chicken with brown rice and fresh vegetables like French beans and broccoli, mushroom risotto with mange tout, baked trout on a bed of steamed vegetables, chicken Caesar salad, raspberry and blueberry medley with yoghurt, poached pears, fruit crumble, grilled peach and plum bruschetta.

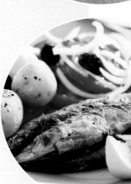

WEEK 2

Recommended changes this week are:

- Change your diet;
- Take vitamin and mineral supplements.

Introduce the pre-conception diet

During the first week it may be a good idea to start buying your new foods if you do not have them in the house already. You do not want to fall into old habits and have the quick Chinese takeaway because you are hungry and do not have anything else to eat. Select foods from the recommended foods listed under carbohydrates, proteins, fats and fibre as well as from the list of foods in the vitamin table. These will form the foundation of your diet for the next three months. Remember it is not about quantity it is about quality; we are not focussing on losing weight. Each as much as you like of these foods when you are hungry and drink plenty of water and herbal teas.

If you find it difficult to think of what to eat at each meal, there are many recipe books available providing healthy options. You are now aware of what foods to eat from the lists provided in this book. Visit your local bookshop and treat yourself to a recipe book that motivates you. It may be a worthwhile investment for those days when you lack imagination or inclination!

Vitamin and mineral supplementation

If you have completed a hair mineral analysis, you will be provided with a detailed supplementation programme of the essential vitamins and minerals that are deficient in your body. This may involve taking one or two tablets with each meal each day. Initially it may appear costly when presented with a bill of between £50–100 each month, depending on what is required. My view is that the money saved from smoking or drinking easily equates to this amount and instead of depleting your body with 'bad' chemicals, you are supplementing with 'good' chemicals.

If you have not completed a hair mineral analysis, it is recommended that you take a good pre-conception vitamin tablet each day. Ideally both partners should take 30 mg zinc, 100 mcg selenium, linseed oil 1000 mg, 50 mg of Vitamin B_6 and B_{12}, 15mg vitamin E, 1000 mg Vitamin C and, for women only, 400 mcg folic acid.

At first it may seem difficult not to grab the occasional pizza or microwave meal but as time passes, the benefits to your health will become apparent and you will not want to return to bad dietary habits. During the last two weeks your body has had a shock, you may have given up smoking and drinking, cleansed the system and now you are eating foods full of vitamins and minerals. Give yourself time to get used to the new you and to incorporate the changes into your daily activities. Don't beat yourself up if you have the odd lapse. The aim of the 3-month pre-conception plan is to give you and your body time to replenish and build up new reserves in order to maximise your chances of conception.

WEEK 3

Recommended changes this week are:

- Continue pre-conception diet;
- Start exercising;
- See your doctor.

Exercise

Now that you are in the swing of making delicious wholefood meals each day, you may feel able to introduce some exercise into your weekly routine if you have not done so already. Yoga, swimming, cycling and walking are all good activities.

Visit the GP

Make an appointment to visit your doctor for both you and your partner to be screened for sexually transmitted diseases. As discussed in step 1, many of the infections are symptomless and can be silently causing damage to your reproductive organs. If either of you tests positive for an infection, a course of antibiotics is sufficient to remove the harmful bacteria and get you back on track to optimising your health for conception. It may take up to two weeks to get the results of the test from your doctor.

WEEK 4

Recommended changes this week are:

- Continue pre-conception diet;
- Try alternative therapies.

Reflexology and acupuncture
I have read countless stories of women who have had some reflexology or acupuncture (see pages 101 and 103) and have become pregnant naturally. The benefits of these treatments are discussed in detail below. Both are good for re-balancing the body's energy system, helping the digestive system and bowels eliminate toxins and increasing your fertility.

When choosing a practitioner, ask for his or her qualifications, how long he or she has been practising and what area of expertise he or she has. Beware of some beauty salons offering these treatments: they tend towards relaxation as opposed to the treatment of ailments. Once you find a reputable practitioner, try to visit him or her at least once per month if possible to maximise your chances of conception.

Congratulations!
You are now at the end of the first month of the pre-conception plan and have made enormous inroads into increasing your chances of getting pregnant. Both you and your partner should congratulate yourselves on getting this far! You may have given up smoking and drinking and will be benefiting from the dietary changes you have made. Your body may feel energised. Exercise and reflexology/acupuncture will be re-balancing your energy flow. You have checked your internal reproductive health for any harmful bacteria. You have taken charge of your fertility, which will hopefully make you feel more confident about your future. Well done! The hard part is over!

MONTHS 2 AND 3

Essentially the next two months are more of the same. Continue the pre-conception diet, take your vitamins, exercise regularly and have a reflexology or acupuncture session. Above all, take time to relax and spend quality time with your partner. Start tracking your ovulation each month and actively have sex at the right time. Good luck!

Ovulation Method

Sometimes called the 'Billings method', the Ovulation Method is covered here for the simple reason that it has helped numerous women identify the ideal time for sexual intercourse and they have subsequently become pregnant. It may sound overly simple but it's surprising how many women are mistaken about the signs of ovulation or do not have obvious signs. Also, because unexplained infertility accounts for 20 percent of infertility cases, could some of these couples be having sex at the wrong time? Women with PCOS (polycystic ovary syndrome) who have irregular menstrual cycles can use this method to help assess if and when ovulation occurs. The Ovulation Method is only concerned with the current cycle and uses reliable natural indications to determine whether a day is infertile, possibly fertile or highly fertile.

How does it work?
Used primarily for natural family planning, the Ovulation Method is based around the fact that ovulation occurs on only one day in each cycle and that the egg lives only 12–24 hours if not fertilised. Sperm, however, may survive up to three days if they are carried in healthy mucus.

When a woman is fertile, mucus is secreted from the glands of the cervix. In a normal menstrual cycle, when menstruation occurs, no mucus is secreted for a few days afterwards. These are 'dry days'; the interior of the vagina is always moist, but the external parts will be dry. This external dryness disappears when mucus levels increase. Soon the amount of mucus increases so that it becomes visible. The mucus alters its appearance over the course of a normal cycle, and, close to ovulation, the mucus becomes clear and slippery and can be stretched without breaking. Women often refer to it as resembling raw egg white. This type of mucus may be present for one day, or a number of days in succession, or it may persist as a lubricative sensation before drying up altogether and becoming cloudy and sticky (see also page 15). The lubricative sensation is the most important indication of maximum fertility and the last day of its presence is called the 'peak'. It is the most accurate indication of ovulation, occurring just before the egg is released from the ovary. Also at this time oestrogen levels peak then fall. The change to dryness or to sticky opaque mucus reflects the rising level of progesterone. At this time in the cycle, intimate sexual contact is most likely to cause conception. Conception can also occur a few days later if the mucus has kept the sperm cells in a healthy state during that time.

Who can benefit from the ovulation method?

All women trying to get pregnant should be interested in knowing their ideal times to conceive. 'Textbook' women have 28-day menstrual cycles and may ovulate between days 14–16 of each month. However, many women have either shorter or longer cycles. This method is ideal as it helps establish a regular pattern of the exact day of ovulation. For example, if you have a 25-day cycle, ovulation may occur between days 11–14 and up until now you may have been actively trying on days 14–16.

Women with anovulatory cycles (do not ovulate regularly) find this method useful. It is easy to assume that we all ovulate each month as nature intended, however, anovulatory cycles are one of the main reasons for infertility. You may not be aware that you are not ovulating each month until you start tracking your patterns using the Ovulation Method. When a women suffers with anovulatory cycles, she will be more aware of the significance of the 'peak' mucus when it appears and be able to actively have sexual intercourse regardless of which day it appears. I have read stories of women who assumed it was safe to have sex towards the end of the month, day 20 onwards, only to become pregnant. Knowing your pattern of ovulation is key to maximising your chances of conception.

The additional benefits of the Ovulation Method are that it does not cost anything to perform, it does not require the administration of drugs and it does not require ovulation or your menstrual cycles to be regular. Other natural methods like the Rhythm Method and Temperature Method have their flaws, as they are concerned with the length and regularity of the menstrual cycle.

Ovulation Method or Ovulation Test Kit?

Ovulation test kits work by detecting an increase in luteinising hormone (LH) in the urine. The LH surge occurs approximately 24–36 hours prior to the release of an egg from the ovaries. You are at your most fertile on the day your LH surge is detected and the day after. Usually two test sticks are provided in a pack and you will need to know your usual cycle length. If you have a normal 28-day cycle, testing is recommended to begin on day 11 and to continue until the LH surge is detected. This may take several test sticks and work out quite expensive, especially if you are testing for ovulation every month until you get pregnant. On the other hand, ovulation test kits are a quick and easy way of letting women know when they are fertile in today's busy world.

Many women opt for the Ovulation Method as it is a no-cost natural way of identifying fertile days and enables them to become more in tune with their bodies. After trying for a baby for many months you may feel like you have become a slave to your menstrual cycle, getting more upset with each passing month. Monitoring it naturally is an ideal way to feel like you are taking charge of your fertility. Both methods are successful in identifying the best time for intercourse and will help to maximise your chances of conception.

Reflexology

A form of complementary therapy, reflexology involves working on the feet or hands to enable the body to heal itself. Following illness, stress, injury or disease, the body is in a state of 'imbalance', and vital energy pathways can become blocked, preventing the body from functioning effectively. Reflexology can be used to restore and maintain the body's natural equilibrium and encourage healing.

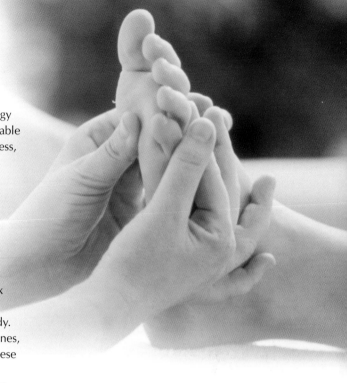

How does it work?

The principle of reflexology is that the reflex points on the feet and hands correspond to organs, glands and structures within the body. Reflexology uses 10 energy paths, called zones, running down the body. If the flow along these zones runs freely, we remain healthy; if, however, the flow is blocked or hindered, an imbalance will occur which, if not treated, will develop as illness or discomfort in the body itself. In the feet, there are reflex areas corresponding to all the parts of the body and these areas are arranged in such a way as to

form a map of the body, with the right foot corresponding to the right side of the body and the left foot to the left side. Sensitive, trained hands can detect tiny deposits and imbalances in the feet, and by working on these points a reflexologist can release blockages and restore the free flow of energy to the whole body. Tensions are eased, circulation is improved and the elimination of toxins is facilitated. This gentle therapy encourages the body to heal itself, often counteracting a lifetime of misuse.

There is now a lot of research into the benefits of reflexology for certain conditions and its practice should not be confused with massage. When a reflexologist talks about 'stimulating' reflexes on the feet and hands, he or she is actually rousing energy that produces a reaction in a specific organ or gland. Many people have experienced significant improvements in their health as a result of the re-balancing of the body's equilibrium.

The idea behind reflexology is not new – in fact it is said to have been used in Egypt, India and China some 5000 years ago, when pressure therapies were used to correct energy fields in the body. But the therapy did not make any real impact in the West until the early 20th century when Dr William Fitzgerald, an ear, nose and

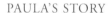

PAULA'S STORY

At 34 I decided that I wanted a second baby but the doctors said that it was 'highly unlikely' that I would ever conceive naturally. But I was determined: my first child was born after four harrowing years of fertility treatment, and this time I wanted to try a natural approach. My doctors were highly sceptical. Undeterred, I booked an appointment with a reflexologist. Two months later I was pregnant. I couldn't believe it! It had taken me four years and four IVF attempts to have Matthew, my first baby. I hadn't had a period in five years, and then, after the first reflexology session, I had one. That in itself was a mini-miracle.

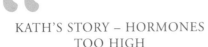

KATH'S STORY – HORMONES TOO HIGH

After three years of trying for our second child we had almost given up hope. Doctors had told me I had a hormone problem, which meant fertility treatment would be a waste of time. I was 40 years old with nothing to lose and had read that reflexology could help with infertility. I had three months of foot massage and, at the end of the course, was delighted to hear my hormone levels had returned to normal. I became pregnant and gave birth to a second son, Fraser, five months ago. While doctors insist there is nothing to prove the complementary therapy was responsible, I'm sure it worked. I was told that there was no point in attempting IVF treatment because it would be a waste, so I would have to resign myself to the fact that we couldn't have another baby. A hormone test, which indicates if a woman is entering the menopause, showed my levels were too high, suggesting my ovaries had stopped producing enough oestrogen, which controls the reproductive cycle. To become pregnant I needed a hormone rating of 10 or below but mine was above 25. Following reflexology, however, it dropped to below eight. The effect of the reflexology was amazing. It seemed to relax me so much. I became pregnant quite quickly and everything went smoothly. The doctors never admitted that the reflexology had anything to do with it but I have no doubt at all.
(Femail.co.uk – 25th March 2003)

throat specialist, became interested in zone therapy, which provided the foundations for reflexology.

Reflexology has traditionally been used in conjunction with conventional fertility therapies to help women become pregnant. However, it is the use of reflexology exclusively to treat infertility that is generating much interest. There are numerous stories of women who have only had reflexology treatment and subsequently become pregnant. The medical profession is still apprehensive and more research is needed in this field to show its benefits.

Who can benefit from reflexology?

Reflexology can help factors that play a part in preventing conception such as blocked tubes, chlamydia and endometriosis, which all affect your ability to conceive. It brings people into balance, helps hormones perform better, relieves stress and promotes lymphatic circulation. Fertility is reliant upon the secretion of appropriate hormones that target reproductive organs in the body. A good reflexologist will pay particular attention to the pituitary gland reflex for the balance of hormone levels within the body, and will also use thumb-walking and pinpoint techniques to stimulate the reproductive system reflexes.

However, it is important to understand that reflexology will not work for everyone. For example, if you have been told you cannot have a baby due to physical reasons, it may not help you get pregnant but it will help re-balance your body and relax you. For women with unexplained infertility and/or hormonal imbalances it is certainly worth a try.

What happens during treatment?

When first visiting a reflexologist, a detailed medical history will be taken. You will be seated in a reclining chair and asked to remove your shoes and socks. The practitioner will initially examine your feet before commencing with the precise massage movement. He or she will apply firm pressure using the sides and end of the thumb. All areas on both feet will be massaged. Areas corresponding to parts of the body that are out of balance, will feel uncomfortable or tender

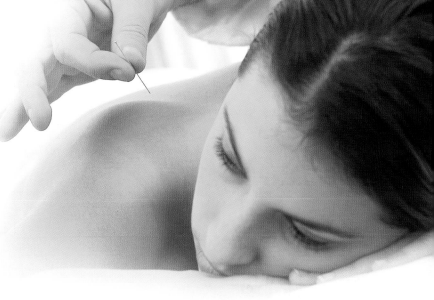

when massaged, and the degree of tenderness will indicate the degree of imbalance. Foot sensitivity varies from person to person; a good reflexologist will know how much pressure to apply and how to interpret the feeling.

The full treatment can last up to an hour and at the end of a session, your feet should feel warm and you will feel relaxed. The number of treatments required will vary depending on the condition being treated.

Following treatment, you may feel tired or completely revitalised, it depends on you. Some people's symptoms get worse before they get better: this can happen if you are fighting an infection or overcoming a painful condition. However, if treatment is correctly applied, these reactions should not be severe.

What the research shows

Up until now, research has been thin on the ground. One study in 1994 by the Danish Reflexologist's Association found that, of 61 women under 35 who had been trying to get pregnant for more than two years, 15 percent became pregnant within seven to eight months of receiving regular reflexology sessions. Of two-thirds of the women who had menstruation problems, 77 percent experienced a significant improvement, with the majority totally getting rid of the problems. Three-quarters of all the women reported improvements in other ailments such as: muscle tension, indigestion, poor circulation and general imbalance.

More research is needed to gain a better understanding of how reflexology can benefit infertile couples. For now, there is an increasing amount of anecdotal evidence from women who became pregnant through reflexology. It assisted me in reducing my high hormone levels and helped regulate my menstrual cycle so that I could start IVF treatment. It is certainly worth a try to see how you may respond to the treatment.

Acupuncture

Acupuncture is a non-invasive complementary form of medicine, which helps re-balance the body to gain optimum health. Practised for more than 3,000 years, this form of Chinese medicine is used as the primary form of health care by over one quarter of the world's population. In 1979, the World Health Organisation detailed over 40 diseases that could be successfully treated with acupuncture, including breathing and digestive problems, disorders of the nervous system and menstrual problems. Acupuncture treatment has helped to regulate menstrual cycles, to improve sperm health and helped couples to conceive healthy babies.

How does it work?

The Chinese believe that the mind and body are inextricably linked. Any imbalance in the flow of energy around the body directly affects its functioning. For example, a person who worries excessively may suffer from irritable bowel syndrome due to the increased mental activity affecting the functioning of the digestive system. Acupuncture treatment focuses on treating the whole person and increasing a person's overall wellbeing.

In traditional Chinese medicine, it is believed that energy, called 'chi', flows along invisible energy channels called 'meridians' which are linked to internal organs. Inserting fine needles at

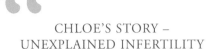

CHLOE'S STORY – UNEXPLAINED INFERTILITY

For more than three years, my husband and I struggled with unexplained infertility. We underwent every available medical test and turned to a series of increasingly drastic fertility treatments. When IVF and two subsequent frozen embryo cycles failed, we began to wonder if we would ever be blessed with children of our own. Then I heard about acupuncture as a potential option.

Initially, I was sceptical. Why hadn't we heard about it before? Would it really work? How could it work when everything else had failed? I did some investigation and found that every Western medical professional I asked about acupuncture told me that it did work. Not wanting to get my hopes up, I jokingly referred to this new style of treatment as my 'witch doctor phase'. Still, I stalled a bit. I visited a naturopath and made arrangements to begin a much lower level assisted therapy than I'd been on before. After another disappointment, I finally went for acupuncture. I was in the middle of an IUI cycle, but the acupuncturist was very comfortable supporting this Western therapy with her treatment. Almost immediately, my body felt different after the treatments. And you could have knocked me over with a feather when I discovered I was pregnant just a few weeks later. Clearly, not everyone will experience such immediate results. I fully expected to undergo at least six months of treatment. But the bottom line for my husband and me is that we're finally going to be parents. And I am absolutely convinced that if I hadn't gone for acupuncture treatment, I wouldn't be decorating a nursery right now.

specific acupuncture points along various meridians can increase or decrease the flow of energy. There are 12 main meridians along which energy flows in the body and 365 acupuncture points. When the body is healthy and balanced, the energy flows freely through the meridians; however, if the energy becomes blocked or weakened, a physical or mental illness can occur.

The reason for a part of the system not functioning effectively may lie elsewhere. The most common diagnosis is a combination of liver energy stagnation, kidney energy deficiency, blood stagnation, blood deficiency, spleen energy deficiency and/or dampness. In Chinese medicine, the kidney is the key organ responsible for reproduction. The first step for a woman is to regulate her menstrual cycle and deal with any abnormalities associated with it. Male infertility is usually due to a combination of kidney yang/yin/chi deficiency. Acupuncture can effectively treat these conditions, resulting in increased sperm count and motility.

Who can benefit from acupuncture?

Acupuncture has also been known to increase fertility by restoring the body's natural equilibrium and maximising the conditions for conception. More specifically, acupuncture is said to increase blood flow to the reproductive organs, stabilize hormone levels and increase ovarian function.

Acupuncture can be used alone to treat functional infertility problems in both men and women. Conditions like irregular ovulation, raised hormone levels and unexplained infertility can all benefit from treatment. Men with low sperm counts, varicoceles, poor sperm motility and erectile difficulties also benefit.

If you require conventional methods like IVF to get pregnant, the good news is you can still have acupuncture treatment. Research has shown that when you combine IVF treatment with acupuncture, the rate of pregnancy increases from 26 to 43 percent.

Initial examination

During the initial consultation the acupuncturist will spend a lot of time trying to gain an accurate

"

ROSIE'S STORY – ACUPUNCTURE AND IVF

I wanted to share my good news with you! I am expecting our new baby! I am 38, soon to be 39, years old. I am very thankful for acupuncture, Chinese herb tea and advice that I received. Last January I decided to 'tweak' my body into optimal fertility. Through acupuncture and the herbal tea I know my body was enhanced for receiving our pregnancy. There was a possibility of miscarriage, and I know that having undergone treatment, I was calm and knew I was doing everything possible for a healthy baby. Acupuncture also helped with my asthma and in many other ways. I have referred several girlfriends for acupuncture treatment, some of whom were told that their chances of getting pregnant were slim. One now has a healthy 1½-year-old and the other is newly pregnant.

When my husband and I first started trying for a baby I thought I would get pregnant immediately. After all, everything in my life had worked on a schedule and I believed that pregnancy would be no different. After three months of 'trying' I started to get a bit concerned and began charting my cycles and taking my basal body temperature every morning. It turned out my cycles were very regular and I ovulated the same time every month. After a few more months with no pregnancy, I then started using ovulation predictor strips; it wasn't long before I was timing my ovulation down to a 12-hour period. My husband and I timed things just right month after month, after month – but no pregnancy.

Our experience was extremely emotionally painful. Why was everything seemingly perfect with my cycles and yet no baby? All tests on both my husband and I were normal so there was no explanation for our infertility. I became obsessive about trying everything I could to get pregnant – special diets, exercise, no exercise, chiropractor, prayer (lots!), taking holidays, yoga, stress counselling, etc., yet still no baby. Finally, out of sheer desperation, we resorted to Clomid (5 rounds) and then intrauterine insemination three times. Still nothing worked.

We decided that since I was age 38 we had no further time to waste and that IVF was in order. I had done a great deal of research on internet discussion groups around infertility and discovered that many women who were successful in IVF treatment did so with acupuncture. Although I was initially quite sceptical, I knew in my heart that unless I had tried absolutely everything that I would feel really bad if the IVF was unsuccessful.

The result was that I felt very relaxed and very positive after each and every treatment. When it came time for my IVF, I received the necessary treatments at the specific times necessary to optimise success. The IVF clinic transferred three embryos. Two weeks later we received the great news – I was pregnant!!

I delivered a very healthy baby girl in March 2004. I fully attribute our success to the specialized acupuncture. Although many will likely say that our daughter was the result of the IVF and nothing more, I have to disagree. Many of the friends I have met online have had to do two or more IVF cycles to get pregnant and there are still many who are not pregnant from IVF. During our IVF cycle I only produced four eggs, which I thought meant inevitable failure of the treatment considering the odds. Those four eggs, however, turned out to be very high quality and produced four top quality embryos. It is this embryo quality that I fully attribute to my acupuncture treatments. One of those embryos is now my beautiful sweet daughter who I love more than anything in this world.

My message to anyone reading this is I know acupuncture can seem like another added expense and use of your valuable time, especially as the cost and time required with IVF is so great, but this is the one area where you can optimise your chances of success.

diagnosis. This consists of four types of examinations, which are asking, looking, listening and smelling, and touching.

Asking During the initial consultation detailed information about your health will be gathered including any pain or symptoms, past illnesses, pattern of menstrual cycle, eating habits, reasons for infertility (if known), lifestyle and overall health. The acupuncturist may ask questions about your relationship with your partner, parents and any significant changes in your life – like moving house.

Looking The acupuncturist will turn his or her attention to your appearance. Are your eyes sparkly? What colour is your face? Is your tongue pink? Does it have a coating? If so, what colour? Different parts of the tongue relate to different body organs. The acupuncturist may draw a diagram to monitor the progress over subsequent treatments.

Listening and Smelling The acupuncturist will carefully listen to you speaking, assessing the tone of your voice and how you express yourself. Breathing patterns are also important as they may indicate an imbalance in the body. It may sound strange, but how you smell can also provide useful information about your internal health. Do you emit a sour smell? Sweet smell?

Touching The final part of the consultation focuses on touching your skin and taking your pulse. The Chinese believe there are six basic pulses, which correspond to specific organs and their function. After entering a relaxed state, the acupuncturist will take a series of pulse readings to ascertain the energy flowing through each point. This is one of the most important aspects of the consultation and may take 20 minutes to complete accurately.

Following the four examinations, the acupuncturist can make an accurate diagnosis and recommend treatment to restore balance within your body.

EVIDENCE OF ACUPUNCTURE'S EFFECTIVENESS

Improvement in sperm quality – A study in Germany showed that acupuncture improved the number and quality of sperm in men who suffered low sperm counts, poor motility and a high number of abnormal sperm.

Improvement of hormone production – The reproductive hormones are released by the pituitary gland in the brain and affect ovarian function. Following acupuncture treatment, many women with irregular menstrual cycles or irregular ovulation have regulated their hormones. Specific attention was paid to the points associated with the hypothalamus-pituitary-ovarian axis.

Raised hormone levels – Older women tend to have more erratic monthly cycles and find it more difficult to conceive. In clinical studies, acupuncture can help normalise levels of FSH, LH, oestradiol and prolactin, increasing the chance of a natural pregnancy. Or if you require IVF due to structural problems, acupuncture will help to lower hormone levels to ensure a better success rate.

Increased IVF success – In cases where couples require IVF, acupuncture before and throughout treatment has shown to increase the pregnancy rate in women undergoing IVF. Forty-two percent of women who underwent IVF treatment and received acupuncture got pregnant, compared to only 26 percent of women who had IVF and no acupuncture. In another study, the pregnancy rates for women undergoing IVF and acupuncture were as high as 51 percent compared to 36 percent of women who had IVF alone. Acupuncture also reduces the risk of miscarriage; only eight percent miscarried compared to 20 percent who did not receive acupuncture.

Treatment

You will lie down and enter a relaxed state before the needles are applied. Many people are initially concerned that it will hurt but most find it painless. There is a slight pinprick when the needle is applied to the acupressure point followed by a tingling sensation. The acupuncturist will use a number of needles depending on the treatment required and will not necessarily place them where you think they should be. The needles are placed along the meridian associated with the organ that is out of balance. The needles may be left for a few minutes or up to half an hour. Sometimes the acupuncturist may warm the needle to stimulate energy to flow to damp areas with a process called 'moxibustion'.

People respond differently to treatment; you may feel sleepy or revitalised at the end of the session. The acupuncturist will recommend how many sessions will be required to bring your body back into a state of balance and how to maximise your fertility. Improvements may be seen after only three to four sessions.

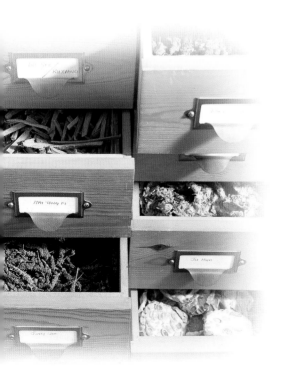

Herbal Medicine

A non-invasive form of complementary treatment, herbal medicine uses the healing powers of plants, flowers, trees and herbs to treat an illness or condition. As with other holistic treatments, herbal medicine does not treat the symptoms but works on the person as a whole to bring the body back into a state of equilibrium. Herbalists will use active ingredients in plants to improve a condition while today's orthodox doctors will use synthetic forms.

Herbal medicine has been practised since ancient times and the World Health Organisation (WHO) estimates that worldwide herbal medicine is three to four times more commonly practised than conventional medicine. Chinese herbal medicine is part of a larger healing system called Traditional Chinese Medicine (TCM), which includes herbal medicine, acupuncture, massage, dietary advice and exercise. Herbal medicine and acupuncture are often used together to re-balance the body's energy meridians and improve a person's fertility.

How does it work?

The theory is that a balance of two opposing forces of energy, called yin and yang, sustains every living thing. Together, they make up the life essence called chi, energy that flows through the body via invisible channels called meridians. Half of certain organs and meridians are governed by yin and the other half by yang. When yin and yang are out of balance in the body, this causes a blockage of chi and a subsequent illness. Yin and yang imbalances can be caused by stress, pollution, poor diet, and emotional upsets or infection. For diagnostic purposes, yin and yang are further subdivided into interior and exterior, hot and cold, deficiency and excess.

Herbs and plants contain active ingredients which, when harnessed correctly, can be used to treat the underlying cause of an imbalance. Many herbs are in common use, such as ginger, which is taken to avoid sickness and nausea, especially morning sickness. Other everyday herbs include garlic, which helps to reduce high cholesterol levels, Gingkbo biloba, which helps

MARY'S STORY

I was in my mid thirties when I started trying to conceive. After a year of trying I visited my GP who arranged tests. During an x-ray examination (HSG) it was discovered that both of my tubes were blocked. With no history of pelvic inflammatory conditions or previous sexually transmitted diseases, the cause of this blockage was unknown. I was advised that there was nothing that could be done to unblock the tubes and that IVF was my only option.

Both my husband and I were unhappy at going through IVF and therefore decided to explore the alternatives. I went see an acupuncturist and herbalist.

My menstrual cycle was erratic and painful. I spotted for several days before my period and was very premenstrual for over a week each month. As the most important barrier to conception was the tube blockage, the practitioner focused on this.

With a combination of herbal medicine and a little acupuncture, we attempted to flush out the uterus. Within three cycles, I felt considerably better, the menses had changed dramatically and on the fourth cycle I booked myself in for an HSG again. Both tubes now were found to be clear. I continued taking the herbs and having acupuncture to regulate my cycle and within another four months I was pregnant. I am the proud mother of a little baby girl, Jess.

important that the herbal medicines follow the natural rhythms of the woman's cycle. During your period, the movement of blood is emphasised so that your body can clear out its old uterine lining thoroughly, making room for a fresh layer. Immediately after your period, the blood is nourished so that your body can replace what has been lost. Around ovulation time, Yin is supplemented to promote the growth of the new egg, and, following ovulation, Yang is supplemented to give energy for the process of fertilisation and implantation in the uterus. By following a woman's natural cycle, herbal medicines can help in each part of that cycle, correcting for irregularities that may be causing problems with fertility.

Once you become pregnant, your herbalist may wish you to stop taking the remedy.

Who can benefit?

The main causes of infertility in women are hormonal and structural and in men are attributed to poor quality and quantity of sperm. Herbal treatment can correct hormonal imbalances and increase the production of the female hormones and the production of the sperm.

Herbal medicine and acupuncture often go hand in hand as treatments. Your practitioner will decide after the initial consultation the most effective way forward.

Vitex

This herb is prescribed to women who have a shortened second half of their menstrual cycles, known as luteal phase defect, and high levels of the hormone prolactin. In one trial, 48 women (aged 23 to 39) who were diagnosed with infertility took vitex once daily for three months. Seven (14.5 percent) women became pregnant during the trial, and 25 (52 percent) of the women experienced normalised progesterone levels, which may increase the chances for pregnancy.

improve depression, and milk thistle, which detoxifies and cleanses the liver. The skill of the herbalist lies in knowing the properties of each herb and being able to mix a remedy specifically tailored to each person's need. Most remedies contain a number of herbs, which work in synergy to produce the required effect.

In treating female infertility, it is extremely

Herbal medicine can also be safely used in conjunction with conventional methods like IVF to maximise the chance of conception. The herbs will improve the health of the reproductive system so that when pregnancy does occur, your body becomes strong enough to carry the baby full term and less prone to miscarriage.

There are many practising herbalists, however, and it is important to find a practitioner who specialises in male and female infertility and is able to combine the treatment with acupuncture, if necessary. The National Institute of Medical Herbalists is a good place to enquire about a practitioner in your area, details can be found under 'useful addresses' on page 157.

What happens during treatment?

The initial consultation will last about an hour. During this time the herbalist will gather as much information about you as possible including your medical history, your lifestyle, your character, what concerns you may have, sleep patterns, diet and any allergies. In addition, your overall appearance is important; the condition of your hair and skin and how you communicate and move also will be assessed. The herbalist is trying to gain an overall picture of you as an individual and to understand what may be causing the imbalance in your body.

The herbalist will also carry out a physical examination and check your pulse, blood pressure, eyes, mouth, tongue, ears and skin.

Following the consultation the herbalist will recommend a remedy. Remedies can be prescribed in a number of forms and usually contain between 10–15 herbs. Remedies to be taken internally include tinctures, infusions and tablets. Tinctures are made from the concentrated essence of soaked flowers, leaves and roots, and a few drops a day are usually prescribed. Infusions are less concentrated and require boiling the herbs in water for 10–15 minutes to release the natural properties. The herbs are removed and the liquid is drunk. Even though they are referred to as herbal 'teas', most of the mixtures have an unpleasant taste to them. Tablets may be recommended for people who find it difficult to drink the 'tea' or tincture. Remedies can also be applied externally to the

LIZ AND CHARLES'S STORY

We had been trying to conceive for three years. Charles had a low sperm count and I was diagnosed with endometriosis. We had been advised that ICSI would be required for me to become pregnant. The herbalist advised that he could help improve my menstrual cycle but that Charles's sperm count was so low that it would be very unlikely that anything other than IVF would work for us. Charles, however, wanted to try to do as much as possible to improve his sperm quality. He received herbal medicine while I had acupuncture and herbs. My treatment progressed smoothly and my cycle became regular and the pain went. After six cycles, my period was unusually late and, although unexpected, the herbalist persuaded us to take a pregnancy test. It was positive! After a difficult pregnancy fraught with bleeding and pain, which we dealt with, we had a beautiful baby boy!

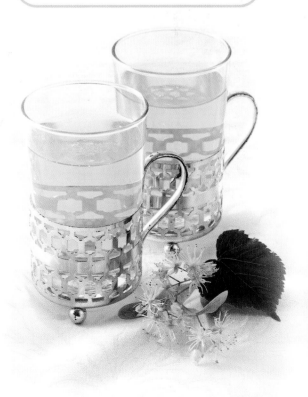

body in the form of creams, ointments, compresses and herbal baths.

Evidence

One study looking at the effectiveness of herbal medicine in helping male infertility concluded that herbal medicine helped improve the condition and in many cases led to the man fathering a child. This occurred in 88 percent of the men with a low sperm count or no sperm at all, 75.5 percent of those with varicocele, 91 percent with abnormalities of seminal fluid and 88 percent in men who had dead sperm. This shows that herbal medicine is a highly effective treatment for male infertility.

REACHING THE SUBCONSCIOUS

A woman's subconscious can alter her body's biochemistry and while she might consciously want a baby, her subconscious may be stopping her from getting pregnant. Hypnotherapy aims to address the underlying worries and concerns.

Hypnotherapy

Hypnotherapy is a complementary form of medicine focusing on the connection between the mind and the body. The practice of hypnosis dates from primitive times when healers would encourage people to cure themselves by planting suggestions of health and well-being during a trance-like state. Today, hypnotherapy is commonly used to treat phobias and a variety of addictions including smoking. Its application to the field of fertility is relatively new and provides a totally different approach to existing outlooks on infertility. For some of you, it may be a radical approach to increasing your chances of conceiving but read on; you will be surprised how the mind can prevent us from conceiving if it wants to.

Hypnotherapy can be used as a stand-alone treatment or in conjunction with other methods to assist you in having a baby.

How does it work?

Hypnotherapy uses hypnosis to access the subconscious mind and deeper aspects of the

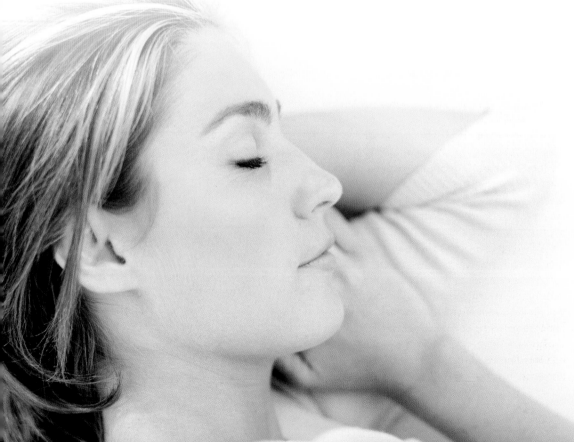

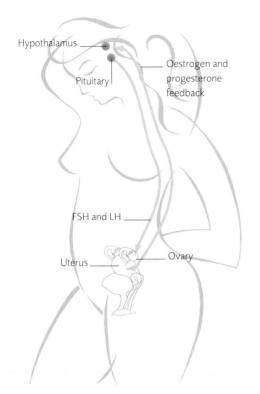

THE MIND-BODY CONNECTION

A complicated feedback system enables the ovary to send information to the brain about oestrogen and progesterone levels, which alerts the hypothalamus gland to stimulate the pituitary to produce follicle stimulating and luteinising hormones, which act on the ovary's follicles.

> ## HELEN'S STORY
>
> After four years of trying to conceive the doctors could find nothing wrong with me or my husband and suggested IVF. We were determined not to go down that road. I felt that if there was nothing physically wrong with me, there must be something else at fault. Shortly into the hypnotherapy programme, I realised that a big part of me did not really want to get pregnant. My career is very important to me. At the back of my mind was the question of whether I could really cope with my business and a child. Also my mother was ill throughout both her pregnancies and had dreadful births. She almost died giving birth to my sister and then I was a breech birth. When you put the package together it is no wonder my mind was playing tricks with my body. I successfully gave birth to my son and quite unintentionally conceived again, five months after giving birth.
> (*Daily Express* January 29 2001)

brain, namely the hypothalamus, the medulla oblongata, and the corpus callosum. It is in these areas of the brain that emotions, memory and instincts lie, as well as our fears and concerns. How many times have you had a 'feeling' that something is not quite right? Or you wake up in the middle of the night with the answer to an issue that has been bothering you for a while? My understanding of hypnotherapy is that it enables deep-rooted thoughts and feelings you may have about pregnancy, childbirth or motherhood to rise to the surface, making you consciously aware of the issues and able to address the problem. Pregnancy may not happen until the problem has been dealt with.

Hypnotherapy works on the basis that there are two states of consciousness – the conscious and subconscious – and these may be at odds with each other. In many cases, the subconscious can alter the body's biochemistry and while a woman might consciously want a baby, her subconscious mind may be stopping her from getting pregnant.

The mind and body are inextricably linked, which is demonstrated not only by complicated feedback systems (see diagram) but also from the effect that stress has on the body. Our mind busies itself with thinking about the problem while the body shows the physical side of stress like a raised heart-rate, raised blood pressure and headache. Hypnotherapy assumes that every thought or sensation experienced in the mind shows itself as some physical change in the body and every physical change will have mental and emotional associations. The reproductive system is no exception.

Who can benefit from hypnotherapy?

It may be a good option if you have any of the following thoughts or feelings:

You are confused about motherhood You care about your career and fear that if you stop work you will lose your identity. You may be anxious not to become like your mother.

You are panicking you are too old Women think their biological age matches their chronological age. It doesn't. We now live longer and take greater care of our health.

You are denying your femininity Perhaps your parents wanted a boy and treated you like one when you were small. You may be subconsciously denying your womb its original function.

You do not think you deserve a child You have low self-esteem, dating from childhood.

You feel ambivalent towards your partner Maybe you fear that you are with the wrong man or that he will leave you.

You feel guilty about having had an abortion There may have been good reasons for the termination but you feel that you are now being punished.

You fear giving birth Some women think they are going to die in childbirth.

Or if you have any of the following physical conditions:

- Unexplained infertility;
- Recurrent miscarriages;
- Polycystic ovaries, endometriosis, anovulatory cycles;
- Inability to conceive after trying for more than 1 year.

These conditions are thought to manifest themselves as a result of psychological barriers a woman may have towards pregnancy, childbirth or motherhood.

There are schools of thought that suggest unexplained infertility is a result of specific factors, which produce unconscious fears and emotions and impair reproductive ability. In addition, factors such as depression, low self-esteem and a sense of failure, can also contribute negatively to the existing situation.

What happens during treatment?

A fertility programme usually comprises 10 one-hour sessions held over two weekly intervals. The initial consultation aims to evaluate your current situation, lifestyle and any health issues in order to determine the best way forward. It also provides you with the opportunity to ask any questions about the treatment to determine if this approach is right for you.

Subsequent sessions involve talking through issues that may be bothering you before you are guided into a trance-like state. The therapist begins hypnosis by encouraging you to relax on a sofa or in a chair. She (or he) talks in a relaxed controlled manner, which encourages you to concentrate on her voice. She asks you to focus on a real or imagined spot in front of you to hold your visual concentration. She may ask you to take several deep breaths, suggesting that with each breath exhaled you feel more relaxed and sleepy. On the final breath you are told to close your eyes. The therapist asks you to imagine a particular scene such as a beautiful white sandy beach and talks you through what you will see and encounter there, encouraging you to use all your senses. She may count you down imaginary steps from ten to one. At this point she may test the depth of your trance by instructing you to perform a simple action such as raising your arm. In unaccustomed subjects it can take up to 20 minutes to get to a level where you are open to suggestions. After several sessions, this

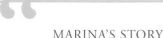

MARINA'S STORY

After four failed IVF attempts I felt a failure. My body was designed to make babies yet all the doctors I visited kept telling me was that it was extremely unlikely I would be able to conceive. Not only did I have to deal with the fact that my fallopian tubes were damaged but the constant negative feedback from doctors made it extremely hard to go on. The hypnotherapy sessions made me realise that I could take charge of my fertility and overcome this feeling of failure. After 10 sessions, I became pregnant naturally. Unfortunately the structural damage in my fallopian tubes meant that at six weeks I miscarried. For the first time I looked on this as a positive occurrence. My body had successfully completed all the difficult biological phases to create an embryo, the beginning of life! This was the turning point for me and never again did I think I might not be able to have a baby. In my case I just needed help getting the embryo from A to B, as the tubes were damaged. So I turned to IVF in the knowledge that this time I could grow a baby all by myself.

reduces significantly as you allow your mind to enter this state. When in the trance you may look like you are asleep but it will not feel like it. Most people feel relaxed, others claim to feel dreamy or feel as if they are floating or watching themselves sleep. You will, however, be aware of what is happening throughout.

Throughout the rest of the session, positive suggestions are made to your subconscious while you visualise yourself in a number of situations with a baby entering into motherhood. Each session's content varies and is tailored to your specific requirements and progress.

In addition to the one-hour session you may be provided with therapeutic audiotapes. The tapes enhance the treatment between sessions and can be listened to as often as possible in the comfort of your home. They provide additional positive reinforcement to the subconscious mind, repeating words of encouragement and asking the body to be effective at a cellular level along the lines of:

'Not only is your body being repaired and revitalised, stores are replenished and recharged, your body is cleansed, blood cells collect all the waste products and transport them away. Your body is functioning more effectively than ever before. You will develop a growing sense of positivity, confidence and sense of control...'

Written assignments may also be given to complement the treatment. To give you an insight into some of the exercises I was asked to do, they involved asking myself 'What do I need in my life to be a happy and fulfilled woman? And what has stopped me in my life from being a happy and fulfilled woman?'

As you begin to peel away the layers to discover the reasons for your infertility you will develop a very intense relationship with your therapist. Your emotional state of mind will fluctuate between 'up' days and those of anger, sadness or guilt. Hypnotherapy is a journey of self-discovery in order to take charge of your fertility.

The evidence

Some therapists have experienced a live birth success rate of 46 percent by using hypnotherapy on their patients. This sounds a promising success rate especially when you compare it to IVF clinics, with an average of 22 percent and even the best at 43.4 percent.

A recent study at Harvard Medical School measured what happened when women who were having difficulty conceiving were given group cognitive behavioural therapy, a technique that replaces negative thoughts with positive ones. During 10 weekly two-hour sessions they were taught how to identify recurrent negative thought patterns and how to separate truth from fear. 55 percent of the women who participated subsequently had a baby, compared to 20 percent of the women who received none.

(ART) Assisted Reproductive Techniques

ART encompasses all the methods in which there is a medical intervention in trying to conceive a baby. The treatments under this umbrella include ovulation induction, intrauterine insemination, in vitro fertilisation and micromanipulation techniques, which increase the chance of fertilisation and implantation such as intracytoplasmic sperm injection and assisted hatching.

In this section, I will look at each treatment, how it works, who can benefit and the success rate you might expect.

IVF is by far the most popular treatment and has recently celebrated its 27th 'birthday'. In the UK, 28,487 couples had IVF in 2003, which resulted in 8544 babies being born, according to the latest figures by the HFEA (Human Fertilisation and Embryology Authority).

One method that has significantly improved fertilisation success rates in the last decade is ICSI (intracytoplasmic sperm injection). Men with sub-optimal sperm can take advantage of this exciting new innovation. Instead of just letting the sperm mix with the egg in a petri dish, the sperm is directly injected into the egg for fertilisation to occur before being placed back into the woman. ICSI now occurs in 44 percent of all IVF treatment in the UK. The medical profession is constantly seeking ways to improve on the overall success rate in order to help couples suffering with infertility realise their dreams of becoming parents.

As a result of the increase in demand for fertility treatment, fertility clinics have sprung up throughout the country. At the last count, there were 85 HFEA-licensed clinics in the UK. Trying to find the right one can be a daunting experience; therefore, this next section has been dedicated to helping you find the right one for you and your partner before discussing each treatment in greater detail.

Clinics

If you and your partner decide on conventional treatments to assist you in getting pregnant, it is important to choose a clinic that will give you the best chance of success and the maximum support. While there are plenty of clinics to choose from, they are not all created equal and the playing field is by no means level. Some clinics are affiliated to a hospital while others are private enterprises with the most sophisticated equipment and clinical expertise. The HFEA publishes rank tables to assist couples in making an informed choice, yet often these are out of date and do not provide enough detail about the success rates for each type of treatment (see also page 118).

Before I advise on choosing a clinic that's right for you, I should like to talk about the common mistakes people make and traps to avoid. I fell into some of these traps because I was naïve and placed my future in the hands of the professionals.

Most of us carefully evaluate and scrutinise items of great importance like a future house or car purchase, yet when the stakes are much higher, all caution and logic may be cast to one side. This is the case with fertility. When it comes to someone providing you with the slightest glimmer of hope of becoming a parent, inevitably you will take a blind leap of faith.

During my IVF treatment I often thought of myself as if I was on some kind of fairground ride. As I approached the fairground, I was filled with excitement and anticipation. Once I got on the ride, I felt a bit anxious about what was going to happen next. As the ride progressed through a few twists and turns, I felt sick, dizzy and wanted to get off before it ended. Once on terra firma again, when the adrenalin rush had subsided, I couldn't wait to get back on to experience it all over again. IVF treatment is an addictive process simply because of your hunger for success. This is why choosing the right clinic from the beginning is one of the most important decisions you will make. If you get it right, you will be on your way to enjoying parenthood.

The Common Traps

Location Some people will choose the nearest clinic to their home. This is understandable as throughout the treatment you will need to be back and forth to the clinic, sometimes several times a day. But it is a mistake to choose a clinic solely on this basis. There are other important factors that must be considered, see below. If you decide that a clinic 200 miles away is a better choice, research the possibility of staying in a local hotel or with friends or taking 3-week holidays from work to focus on your goal.

If your health authority has offered you treatment on the NHS (usually only one cycle), your options may be more limited to the clinics within the authority or immediate area. If you are a 'paying customer' you will have more choice.

Hearsay and recommendation Choosing a clinic solely on the fact that you heard a doctor there was 'good' or you know someone who went there and has had a success is wrong. Sure, it provides you with a place to start but again your research must go beyond this to identify what the clinic can do for YOU. Every couple's circumstances vary and what works for one couple may not work for another. Bear this in mind when researching the types of treatment available at each clinic.

Referral from a GP or gynaecologist After completing your initial investigative tests, your doctor will undoubtedly have a conversation with you about what happens next. So far you

MARINA'S STORY

Throughout my first IVF cycle I was like a sponge absorbing all the information, assimilating facts and figures while trying to ask the right questions. The problem was I did not know what to ask so I listened and took in all the information in good faith.

I leaned heavily on my gynaecologist to help me in understanding the daunting world of infertility. He recommended a clinic that was 30 minutes away and I was delighted because it meant that I could slip out from work if I needed to have blood tests or visit them after work. It was highly convenient.

My first cycle failed because I suffered from OHSS (Ovarian Hyperstimulation Syndrome). I was given too many fertility drugs and not monitored over a holiday weekend, as the clinic was closed. There was no way my body could have accepted live embryos so they were frozen for a later date. I had immediately reduced my chances to about 10 percent.

Unsurprisingly, I chose the same clinic for my second attempt because it was close by and I got on very well with the consultant. But I was overstimulated again and became extremely unwell. More embryos were frozen and I was emotionally devastated.

With hindsight I should have become my own best advocate and done more research. If I had done so, I would have identified that this hospital operated a five-day week and had a very low level of 'live' transfers. Now I know why!

It took me four IVF attempts, thousands of pounds and nearly cost me my marriage until I found the right clinic for us. I had spent six years trying for a baby and was running out of time, for I was 37 years old. But, after one attempt at the right clinic 200 miles away, we have a gorgeous little boy!

have invested all your trust in your GP or gynaecologist and will naturally respect his/her choice of clinic. Often, a doctor's referral may be based on hearsay or anecdotal information or sometimes on casual professional acquaintances. Certainly research your doctor's recommendation but if the clinic does not suit you and your partner, do not feel pressurised into using it.

Cost It is in our nature to seek out a good deal. When it comes to fertility treatment there is no such thing as a good deal. The cost of treatment bears no relation to the clinic's success rate. What does pay off is the time you invest in researching and asking the right questions.

Repeat treatment You may have already completed one cycle of treatment at a chosen clinic and wish to try again. Do not feel under pressure to use the same clinic for your next attempt. If it has not worked the first time, there may be a valid reason for it, such as their opening times, which may be out of your control.

Fast-track clinic choice

Couples have varying approaches to their infertility. Many find their own way and are happy to let fate takes its course. This is a great approach if you have enough reproductive years ahead of you to allow you to learn from your mistakes. However, a quicker approach outlined below will guide you in the right direction.

Questionnaire

The questions are not exhaustive and are in no order of priority. Choose those that you feel will best help you find the right clinic. While they'll help you gain a better understanding of which clinic is right for you, you must do your research and become an expert. The stakes are too high to leave it to chance alone!

Background
- How long has the clinic been established?
- Is there a waiting list for treatment?
- How many treatments are carried out a year?
- Are there any restrictions to treatment at the clinic? (e.g. BMI less than 30, negative screening for AID tests, Hepatitis B and C)
- Does the clinic have a maximum age limit that it will accept to treat?
- What does the clinic do differently than others?
- What is the policy regarding the number of embryos replaced?
- What is the policy on cancelling the treatment if too few or too many eggs develop?

- Does the clinic offer genetic screening for cystic fibrosis or other genetically transmitted diseases?
- What is the clinic's policy for decreasing the risk of ovarian hyperstimulation syndrome (OHSS)?
- How many cycles does the clinic recommend before seeking other treatment options?
- What is the clinic's policy on screening donors?

Success rate
- What is the live birth rate per treatment cycle started, per egg collection, per embryo transfer?
- How many pregnancies resulted in multiple births? Singletons? Triplets?
- How many babies have been born to women aged 30 to 39? 40 and above?
- What percentage of live embryo transfers are carried out versus frozen embryo transfers?

Treatment
- What is the process? How many days will it take? When is the ideal time to start?
- What tests will I need to have before treatment is commenced?
- Why do I need to have each test?
- What are the side effects of the drugs?

Get to know your clinics Allocate time to pore over statistics, research books or find information on the Internet. Telephone a few clinics and ask them key questions about their business. Once you have a shortlist, take the time to visit each one. What kind of environment does it have? How did you feel when you walked in? Are the staff friendly and welcoming?

Evaluate all your options Collate all the information about costs, location, waiting times, success rates, multiple birth rate, etc.

You might like to adopt some kind of rating system, like awarding stars or points. This will give you an overview of the pros and cons of each clinic and help you make an informed decision. There may be one clear winner or you may have to compromise on some factors if the clinics are comparable.

Make the most of your initial consultation Make an appointment to meet your practitioner and his/her team. Ask your questions and ensure you gain a copy of the clinic's patient literature and costs. If you are happy with your decision, you can schedule a date to start your fertility treatment. If not, you may need to revisit your evaluation sheet.

Use the questionnaire To assist you with your enquiries. I've compiled a list of the most useful questions to ask, see below.

- How can I expect to feel?
- How do I administer the drugs?
- Can someone else administer them for me?
- How many times will I have to visit the clinic?
- Does the clinic have embryo storage facilities?
- Does the clinic have access to donor sperm/eggs/embryos?
- Is combined IVF and GIFT treatment offered?
- What is the clinic's multiple birth rate for this treatment?
- What will happen if we achieve pregnancy?
- What tests will you do when I am pregnant? When?
- What will happen if we don't achieve pregnancy?
- How long before you recommend we try again if we are unsuccessful?
- What other treatments does the clinic offer?
- Does the clinic have transport or satellite treatment arrangements with a hospital closer to my home?
- Is the clinic open at weekends?
- Does it offer extended hours?
- Is it open on Bank Holidays?

Cost
- What is the cost of treatment?
- What is the cost of drugs?
- What is the cost of tests?
- What payment methods do you accept?
- How often will we be billed?
- Will there be any additional costs other than those quoted?
- If we use satellite services how will we be expected to pay?
- Can we defer payment until the end of treatment?

Service
- Will we see the same doctor/team members throughout treatment?
- What counselling is available to us as a couple?
- Does the clinic have a patient support group?
- Can I see a woman doctor if I wish?

Live birth rate

All clinics furnish data on their results, generally in the form of charts and graphs. The live birth rate (see page 120) being of most interest to you. Below are examples of what I would consider good data and poor data from clinics and an explanation of what they show and why this is important for judging any clinic's results.

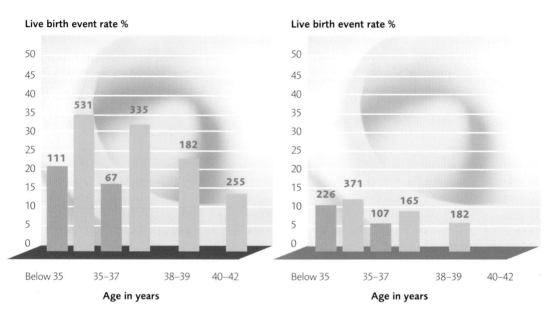

Live birth event rate %

Live birth event rate %

Age in years

Age in years

Live embryo transfers   Frozen embryo transfers

(coloured number= treatment cycles)

CLINIC 1 GOOD DATA

This tells us this clinic has completed 1481 treatment cycles that year, with 88% of the cycles using fresh embryos. The success rate for live transfers in each age group were 35% for below 35-year-olds, 33% in the 35–37-year-olds, 24% in the 38–39-year-olds and 14% in the 40–42-year-olds. Frozen embryos cycles represented 12% of the treatment cycles and the majority were for women under 37 years old. This may indicate that the embryos in women over 37 were not 'good quality' eggs suitable for freezing. If you are over 37, were considering this clinic and wanted the option of frozen embyros, this may be one of your questions to ask during the consultation – 'Why are there no figures for frozen embryo transfers for women over 37?'

CLINIC 2 BAD DATA

This tells us that this clinic has performed 1,051 treatment cycles that year, of which 68% were live embryo transfers. This resulted in a 13% live birth rate below 35 years old, 9% in 35–37-year-olds, 6% in 38–39-year-olds and none in the 40–42-year-olds. These success rates are below the national average. Moreover, when looking at the table of figures that accompanies the graph, it shows that although this clinic had 371 women under 35 start cycles in that year, only 340 went on to have egg collection and out of those only 286 had embryo transfers. That is a high drop-off rate; 85 women did not complete treatment for whatever reason. You may expect between 5–10% of women not responding to treatment but not 29%. This would require more research as to the reasons why.

Live birth event rate %

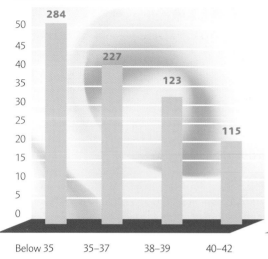

Age in years

Live birth event rate %

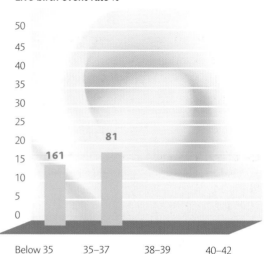

Age in years

CLINIC 3 GOOD DATA

This tells us this clinic has completed a total of 749 treatment cycles in that year of which 99% of the treatments used fresh embryos, which have resulted in some excellent success rates. When looking at the accompanying table it shows that out of the 284 women under 35 starting treatment, 283 had egg collections and 280 went on to have embryo transfers. The below 35 age group provides the highest live birth rate of 58.5%; the 35–37 age group had a 41.4% live birth rate; the 38–39-year-olds had a 33.3% live birth rate, and the 40–42s had a 20% live birth rate. In this particular year it appears the clinic did not complete many frozen embryo transfers (34).

Percentages are not calculated where there are less than 50 cycles, so no graph will show this. Having so few frozen transfers is not a bad thing; it may mean the clinic is very good at managing the ovarian stimulation process to ensure as many women as possible have a live embryo transfer, and this is also reflected in the extremely low 'drop out' rate. (Only 4 women under 35 did not complete treatment.) Live embryo transfers result in significantly higher live birth rates than frozen embryo transfers. In addition, different clinics may have different criteria on which embryos to freeze, for example, one clinic may freeze any remaining Day 3 embryos whereas others may only freeze the embryo if it reaches the blastocyst stage on day 5, as it will be more robust.

CLINIC 4 BAD DATA

This tells us that this clinic may be a small clinic, as it carried out 242 treatment cycles that year. The size of the clinic is not important: how it performs is. I have included this graph as it is curious. Why is there a higher success rate in the 35–37-year-olds compared to women under 35? You would typically expect the graph to be the other way around with the higher success rates in younger women. Again, it is worth asking the questions if you were considering this clinic.

Rank tables explained

The field of infertility is growing at a rapid rate. There are currently 85 fertility clinics in the UK to meet the rising demand for treatment. In 1990 the Department of Health passed the Human Fertilisation and Embryology Act 1990, a year later the Human Fertilisation and Embryology Authority was set up to govern the fertility practices and clinics in the UK. The HFEA's primary task is to license and monitor clinics that carry out IVF, donor insemination and human embryo research.

Each clinic is required to submit its yearly results to the HFEA, who register and collate for the patients benefit. The HFEA *Guide to Infertility* and *Directory of Clinics* is published by the HFEA and should be your first point of reference when choosing a clinic. The guide provides invaluable information about each clinic, what treatment it offers and success rates, that will enable you to compare clinics directly. The guide can also be downloaded from the HFEA website at www.hfea.gov.uk.

Understanding the statistics

Most couples start by looking at the clinic they have been referred to or one that is local to them. This is a great place to start but make sure you compare your chosen clinic with the average national figures for that type of treatment. There is no point using a clinic with a 15 percent live birth rate when a clinic that is an hour away can improve your chances to 25 percent. Do your research, take time to investigate each clinic and look specifically at the following figures in the Guide (see box).

Live birth rate This is the most important statistic to you. We are only interested in how

successful the clinic is in delivering live babies – after all, this is what you want! The live birth rate chart shows the individual clinic's relative success rate for that clinic between different treatment cycles involving fresh and frozen embryos by different age groups. The rate is calculated by dividing the number of live birth events by the number of treatment cycles started. On the previous pages, I include some sample charts provided by HFEA and elucidate the information they provide.

Poor data There are many clinics within the HFEA Guide that do not provide enough statistical data to produce a graph and it therefore appears completely blank. Having no data does not necessarily mean a clinic is a 'bad' one; it may indicate the clinic is relatively new or that less than 50 treatment cycles were carried out in that year. If the one you have chosen appears blank, please contact it to ask the reason why before arranging your initial consultation. You need as much information about your chosen clinic as possible as you do not want to be on your third IVF treatment cycle before realising this clinic is not the one for you. Use the questions on pages 116–17 to guide you.

Percentage of ICSI cycles performed This is another figure that may be of interest to you. Browsing through the guide it is apparent that some clinics only use ICSI (intracytoplasmic sperm injection) in 21 percent of the treatment cycles whereas others use ICSI in 79 percent of their treatment cycles. ICSI, which is discussed here and on page 134, has significantly increased live birth rates, especially in couples with sub-optimal sperm.

One of the most important steps in IVF is egg collection and then fertilising those eggs with the sperm. Sperm quality and quantity are assessed by the embryologist prior to fertilisation. If the sperm are thought to need assistance with fertilisation, ICSI is performed; sperm are injected directly into the egg to bring about fertilisation. If no assistance is required, the egg and sperm will be placed next to each other so the sperm can penetrate the outer shell itself. ICSI significantly improves fertilisation rates and subsequently more embryos are available for transfer back into the womb.

At first glance it appears that the clinic with a 21 percent ICSI rate may have more virile men attending this clinic but it seems unlikely. It may suggest, however, that clinics have thresholds on sperm quality and quantity and a clinic may have tougher parameters; for example, it will select only 'good' or 'excellent' sperm to fertilise on their own. With any sperm below this classification, ICSI will be recommended. Another clinic may only use ICSI with sperm classified as 'poor' to increase the fertilisation rate. If the clinic has a high live birth rate and a high ICSI rate, this suggests that the clinic uses ICSI to improve fertilisation rates, which results in a higher number of live births. It is worth asking the clinic how it approaches the decision and what are its criteria for ICSI.

Other figures of interest These include the number of single births versus multiple births and the drop-off rate, i.e., cycles started in your age group and how many women actually had an embryo transfer. If you are having donor insemination, a summary table details the success rates per age group.

Please bear in mind that the HFEA Guide is one year out of date by the time it is published. Your clinic may have another whole year's data available, which has not yet been published. Contact the clinic to get the latest information. The rank tables are to be used only as a guide; the HFEA cannot tell you which is the best clinic for you, only you can decide. I hope this has helped point you in the right direction but now it is down to you to research, research, research!

THE TECHNIQUES

These include ovulation induction, intrauterine insemination, in vitro fertilization and the micromanipulation techniques of intracytoplasmic sperm injection and assisted hatching.

OI (Ovulation Induction)

Also called ovarian stimulation, OI is usually the first assisted reproductive treatment that women will turn to when seeking help to get pregnant. Of the reasons for infertility in women, 30 percent are due to ovulation disorders. Fertility drugs, which help women achieve ovulation, have proven to be successful. The drugs are inexpensive and can be taken over a 3–6 month period. Research has shown that if pregnancy has not occurred during this time, ovulation induction is unlikely to result in pregnancy and a couple should seek other types of treatment to help them conceive.

How does it work?
Fertility drugs have been developed that help regulate and stimulate ovulation. The most common drugs used for ovulation induction are clomiphene citrate (Clomid), Serophin, Metaformin and Parlodel. They work by fooling the body into thinking oestrogen levels are low. The brain picks up on the signal and responds by increasing the production of FSH and LH, which then stimulates ovulation to occur. In some cases, a woman may release more than one egg a month, however, the risk of a multiple pregnancy occurring is only five percent.

The tablets are taken once a day starting between days 2–6 of the menstrual cycle for a period of five days. The doctor will prescribe the dosage necessary to kick-start ovulation; the lowest dosage is 50 mg. This dosage may be increased in subsequent months if you have not become pregnant. Of women using these drugs, 80 percent will ovulate and 50 percent will conceive.

A maximum period of six months' use is recommended, as there are side effects with continued use. These include headaches, mood swings, hot flushes, breast tenderness, nausea and vomiting. In addition, women may experience enlarged ovaries, ovarian cysts and in rare cases, Ovarian Hyperstimulation Syndrome (see page 60). Your doctor may examine you during your treatment to see how you are responding to the drugs, and to check that ovarian cysts have not developed. Some women report bad side effects while others have none.

Who can benefit?

Ovulatory disorders in women are the second most common cause of infertility after structural causes like damaged fallopian tubes. Women with PCOS (Polycystic Ovarian Syndrome), hormonal imbalances, and irregular or infrequent periods may benefit from this treatment. It may not be suitable for women with premature ovarian failure (early menopause) or effective in women over 40, or those with blocked or damaged fallopian tubes.

Evidence

Clomiphene citrate results in ovulation in 75–90 percent of women with PCOS. Of those that ovulate, 60–70 percent conceive with 40–50 percent resulting in live births.

IUI (Intrauterine insemination)

Otherwise known as artificial insemination, IUI involves inserting sperm into a woman's uterus at the time of ovulation to meet the egg and fertilise it. For many couples, IUI tends to be less invasive and less expensive than other methods of assisted conception. If you've been trying to conceive for quite some time and are considering what to do next, intrauterine insemination is one option you should consider.

How does it work?

Essentially IUI gives sperm a head start in trying to fertilise an egg by placing them directly into the uterus in large quantities. A normal ejaculate contains up to 300 million sperm, of which only one million reach the cervix, 200 reach the fallopian tube and one fertilises an egg. IUI increases the number of sperm that reach the fallopian tube to maximise the chances of conception.

When a couple decide to have IUI, they will be offered the option of having IUI using the woman's natural cycle in which only one egg is released, or increasing the number of eggs released by using fertility drugs. Stimulated IUI cycles tend to have higher success rates than un-stimulated cycles. This is thought to be due to the fact that women may have an underlying ovulatory disorder that can be overcome with the use of stimulation drugs. Or, it could just be that more eggs and more sperm will increase the chances of fertilisation taking place.

A natural cycle The woman is monitored with a blood test and scan between days 12–15 of her menstrual cycle to pinpoint the natural surge in LH (luteinising hormone), which indicates ovulation is about to take place. Timing is essential to the success of IUI; six hours either side of ovulation is thought to be the ideal time. The egg survives for a maximum of 24 hours after it is released. The man provides a sample of sperm, which is assessed, prepared and washed prior to being placed into a very fine catheter. The catheter is placed inside the uterus. Sperm can live up to five days if the mucus is healthy.

Stimulated cycle Fertility drugs, such as clomid tablets, are administered to increase the number of eggs produced. One or two blood tests and ultrasound scans will confirm the development and size of the follicles as well as a woman's readiness for ovulation and insemination. When the time is right, she will be injected with the hormone HCG (human chorionic gonadotropin), which causes the egg to be released from the follicle 36 hours later. The prepared sperm are inserted into the catheter and placed in the upper part of the womb cavity.

Who can benefit?

Couples who have been trying to conceive for a while may choose IUI initially, as it is less invasive and less expensive than IVF. You may wish to try IUI over a three- to six-month period before discussing other options with your doctor. It can help to improve the chances of conception for couples with unexplained infertility, women with endometriosis and men with mildly reduced sperm quality. However, IUI is not suitable for women with blocked or damaged fallopian tubes or poor egg quality, or those who have experienced premature menopause or are aged 40 or over, or for men with a very poor sperm quality. Success rates for IUI are between 10–15 percent per cycle. The success rates depend on the age of the woman, the quality of the sperm and how long the couple have been infertile.

Evidence

Research has shown that the higher the sperm count, the greater the chance of a successful pregnancy with IUI. Some research suggests that if the sperm count is low, IVF with ICSI would be a more successful treatment.

One study of 332 couples who underwent 1115 cycles of IUI resulted in an overall pregnancy rate of 18.7 percent. Of the pregnancies, 16 percent occurred in the first three treatment cycles and this increased to 26.9 percent by the sixth cycle. The research concluded that lower pregnancy rates with IUI resulted if the woman was older than 39 or the total motile sperm count per insemination was less than one million.

IVF (In Vitro fertilisation)

This is the most popular method of assisted conception and involves fertilising a woman's eggs outside her body under controlled laboratory conditions and replacing the embryos back into the uterus (for the process, see also pages 128–29).

IVF was initially designed as the treatment for women with irreparable fallopian tube damage. It is now frequently used as a treatment option for couples with other types of fertility problems such as sub-optimal sperm, ovulatory disorders, endometriosis and unexplained infertility.

With IVF, a couple can use their own eggs and sperm, frozen embryos, or egg and sperm donated from anonymous donors. According to the HFEA's most recent figures (2003), of couples who undergo IVF, 74.8 percent use their own fresh eggs and embryos, 19.3 percent use frozen embryos from their own eggs, 4.4 percent have fresh embryos from donor eggs and 1.5 percent use frozen embryos from donor eggs. Typically, fresh embryos are used in the first treatment cycle, while the remaining embryos may be frozen and used in subsequent treatments. Only a small percentage use egg donors.

The risk of multiple births increases with IVF treatment. The Code of Practice governed by the HFEA changed in 2004 to state that no more than two embryos should be transferred in any one treatment cycle for women under 40 and no more than three embryos in a cycle for women aged 40 and over. In 2003, 75.8 percent of women who became pregnant with IVF gave birth to one child, 23.6 percent to twins and 0.5 percent to triplets.

All fertility clinics tend to follow the same IVF process but apply their own subtle variations to the process to achieve their success rates. Success rates do vary widely throughout the country – from 10 percent to 58 percent live birth success rate – but the average is 25–30 percent. This means that over three-quarters of couples may be unsuccessful in conceiving a child with IVF. From my experience, it is how the clinic tailors the process to each couple's situation that distinguishes a successful clinic from a less successful one. No two women respond the same way to the fertility drugs and continually tweaking the process throughout the treatment cycle seems to be the main factor in maximising a couple's chance of pregnancy. Nobody likes to be treated like a number and made to feel she is on the same production line as everyone else, which often happens!

How does it work?

A woman is stimulated to produce multiple eggs with fertility drugs. When the eggs are mature, they are collected and placed in a test tube with the prepared sperm to encourage fertilisation under controlled conditions. The resulting

% success rate

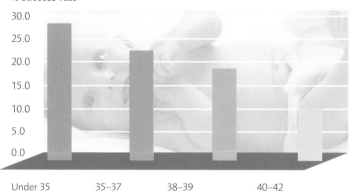

30.0
25.0
20.0
15.0
10.0
5.0
0.0

Under 35   35–37   38–39   40–42

Age in years

AVERAGE SUCCESS RATE FOR IVF USING FRESH EMBRYOS
Fresh embryos produce a much greater chance of success compared to frozen embryos.

embryos are placed back into the uterus with a very fine catheter to implant and develop. This is a simplistic way of describing a complex process in which many factors have to come to play at exactly the right time to ensure success.

The IVF process can be divided into several key stages:
• Preparation
• The initial consultation
• Fertility investigations
• Confirmation of treatment and protocol
• Fertility drugs and ovarian stimulation
• Egg collection
• Embryo transfer
• Pregnancy test

The table opposite highlights the sequence of events and when each stage takes place. I have assumed that week 1 is the date of the initial consultation. Take note of how long after the consultation it may take before ovarian stimulation is started. With my first IVF treatment, I was naïve in thinking that I would start straight after my consultation, and did not realise the clinic needed to complete all these tests beforehand, many of which were at specific times of the month. As a result, I became incredibly impatient as I was mentally ready to start then and there!

Don't hesitate to ask questions throughout the treatment if you do not understand what you are being asked to do. Many couples undergoing treatment feel that they are no longer in charge of their fertility and it is now up to their doctors

to achieve success. While it is true that you do need medical assistance, I believe it is very important to remain in charge of your fertility by understanding what is happening at each stage, becoming fully involved and questioning reasons behind decisions that are made. You will feel less stressed, more in control and hopefully increase your chance of pregnancy. Below, I consider each stage of the IVF process in turn.

Preparation
I believe preparation is the key to a successful IVF treatment cycle. More specifically, choosing the right clinic and preparing yourself physically and mentally for what lies ahead.

Choosing the right clinic I have mentioned this several times throughout the book as I truly believe a lot of the success is down to finding the right clinic for you and your partner. A whole section (see pages 114–120) has been dedicated to helping you find the right clinic and knowing what questions to ask. Do your research and question all the time.

Physical preparation Your body will need to be in optimum condition throughout the IVF treatment cycle. IVF is a very demanding process. Physically you are subjecting your body to powerful drugs, which have well-documented side effects. Many women equate it to having premenstrual tension a thousand times over.

To gain optimum health, follow the wholefood diet plan for a few months prior to

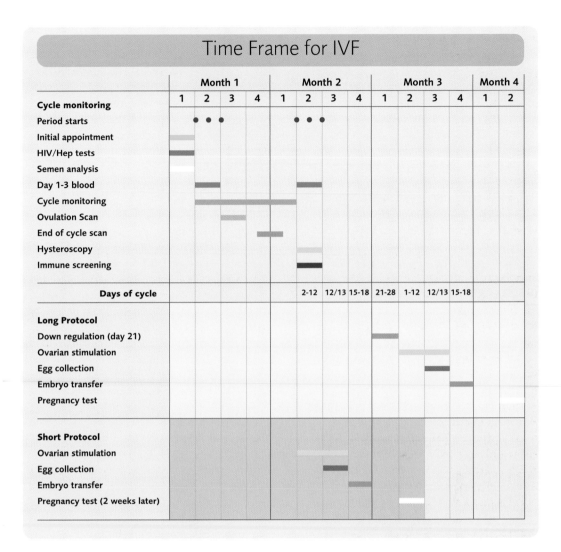

Time Frame for IVF

	Month 1				Month 2				Month 3				Month 4	
	1	2	3	4	1	2	3	4	1	2	3	4	1	2
Cycle monitoring														
Period starts														
Initial appointment														
HIV/Hep tests														
Semen analysis														
Day 1-3 blood														
Cycle monitoring														
Ovulation Scan														
End of cycle scan														
Hysteroscopy														
Immune screening														
Days of cycle					2-12	12/13	15-18	21-28	1-12	12/13	15-18			
Long Protocol														
Down regulation (day 21)														
Ovarian stimulation														
Egg collection														
Embryo transfer														
Pregnancy test														
Short Protocol														
Ovarian stimulation														
Egg collection														
Embryo transfer														
Pregnancy test (2 weeks later)														

treatment to ensure you are eating all the essential nutrients necessary for pregnancy. A three-month plan can be found on pages 94–99. Take a pre-conception vitamin tablet, which contains folic acid. If you are over- or underweight according to your BMI (Body Mass Index), aim to lose between 5–10 percent of your weight before starting treatment. Keep yourself active through swimming, yoga, walking and cycling. Any bad habits like smoking, drinking and drug taking should have been stopped the moment you decided to try for a baby. It takes time for the body to rid itself of these toxic chemicals and cleanse itself.

Complementary treatments like reflexology and acupuncture work extremely well in preparing your body for IVF. These treatments can safely be used alongside IVF to maximise your chances of pregnancy. Research has shown that acupuncture can increase your chances of successful IVF by 10 percent. I use reflexology as I respond very well to the treatment and have a good relationship with my therapist. She knows my medical situation and is able to arouse the right energy meridians at the right time. Spend time reading about how complementary treatments can enhance IVF and try to find a therapist that specialises in infertility.

Mental preparation You are effectively shutting down your normal menstrual cycle and becoming menopausal and to do so, fertility drugs have to send powerful messages to your brain. Headaches, hot sweats, irritability and moods swings are common side effects. Simon and I have been through the IVF process many times and each time we are surprised at how quickly these symptoms appear. We are never ready for the mood swings. One minute I'm happily bumbling along and the next I turn into a raving lunatic – shouting, screaming, angry and aggressive. We now understand that it is part of the process and try to anticipate when it may hit us. If this happens to you, make sure you explain to your partner that it's not you; it's the fertility drugs and it's only short term. Many men may run a mile if they do not understand what is happening! Ensure your relationship is on an even keel before starting. You will need all the emotional support available to get through any difficult moments.

I also advise you to try to eliminate all stressful situations from your life for the next few months if possible. For example, there is little point in having IVF if you are in the process of moving house. You need all your attention to be focused on this one very important task. If you have a demanding job it may be worth confiding in your boss that you are having IVF treatment, in order to get less pressure for a short period of time. Many women take a holiday for the final two weeks of the process to maximise their chances of success.

The paperwork

There are several forms that need to be completed prior to embryo transfer, many of which have essential legal implications. Take your time to run through these forms with your partner and understand them. For example, how many embryos do you wish to replace? Do you wish your sperm or eggs to be used in treating others? Or used for research? Do you wish to freeze any viable embryos after transfer, if so, for how long? If you die or become mentally incapacitated do you wish your sperm/eggs or embryos to be allowed to perish? Or to continue in storage for your partner to use? The forms required by the clinic and HFEA include:

- **HFEA** (00)6 Form for consent to storage and use of sperm and embryos
- **HFEA** (00)7 Form for consent to storage and use of eggs and embryos
- Consent forms for IVF/ICSI/GIFT
- Consent form for embryo transfer

Initial Consultation

You have done all your research to find the right clinic for you and your partner and are now mentally ready to start treatment. Unfortunately, as the number of people seeking IVF treatment has risen over the years, most clinics in the UK have a waiting list. My advice is to make an appointment as soon as you have made the decision to have IVF; you could be waiting three months or more. The reality is that you have been actively trying for a baby for a while now, completed fertility testing and will be feeling impatient. You want a baby as soon as possible. It's incredibly hard to wait another few months; be patient and do not make the mistake of finding another clinic with a shorter waiting list just so you can start right away. There is a reason why your research has led to a particular clinic!

The initial consultation typically lasts an hour, during which time essential information is gathered about you and your partner. Ensure that you have all the necessary dates and details to hand. You may have been sent a form to complete prior to the consultation. Information required usually includes: name and address of your referring doctor, how long you have been trying to conceive, any previous fertility investigations/treatment and medical history. More specifically, how long your menstrual cycle is, any problems observed, date of last period, abnormal smear test results, any previous pregnancies/miscarriages, serious illnesses or genetic disorders in the family, plus the essential lifestyle questions – smoking, drinking, allergies. Use your time wisely and have your questions about the treatment and clinic ready so you can leave happy with all the information. The questionnaire on pages 116–17 will help you.

Be sure the potential cost of treatment is explained fully to you at this stage: you do not want the stress of any additional costs at the end of the treatment when you are trying to relax. Most clinics charge between £2500–£3000 for IVF treatment, which includes the consultant's and operating theatre's cost. Fertility drugs, blood tests and scans tend to be charged for separately. Find out how your clinic charges, how often you can make payments and what the expected cost may be. In my experience, there is a huge benefit in having regular blood tests and scans, the down side is the cost! As an example, during my last IVF treatment I had 13 blood tests over the 10-day period, which alone cost £390.

The final part of the consultation is the assessment of the male partner and completion of a semen analysis. A comfortable room may be provided to collect the semen. Within a few days, the clinic will provide you with feedback on the semen analysis and highlight any potential issues. At this stage it may become apparent that in order to successfully fertilise the egg additional techniques like ICSI (intracytoplasmic sperm injection) may be required to help increase the fertilisation rate. Details of what is assessed during a semen analysis can be found on page 72.

During or after the consultation, the clinic will confirm verbally or in writing that it is able to help you and your partner. This is great news; you are on your way to trying for a baby. The next stage is to complete further investigations and blood tests prior to commencing stimulation.

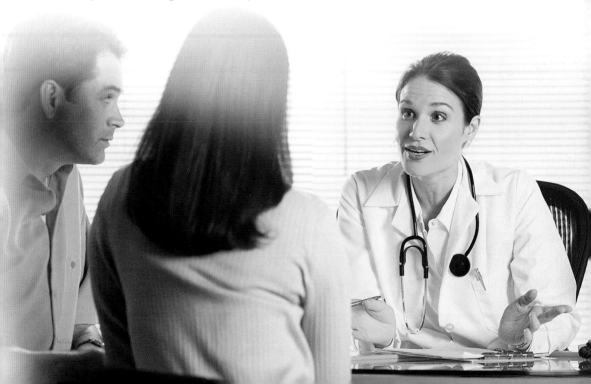

The process of IVF

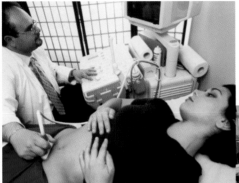

STAGE 1: OVARIAN STIMULATION
Fertility drugs stimulate the ovaries to produce several eggs over a 10–14 day period. Regular monitoring determines the growth and development of the eggs within the follicles and the readiness of the uterine lining for implantation.

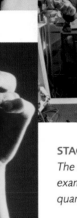

STAGE 2: EGG COLLECTION
The eggs are extracted under anaesthesia and examined microscopically by an embryologist. The quantity and quality of the eggs is established.

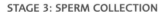

STAGE 3: SPERM COLLECTION
A sample of semen is provided and examined microscopically to assess the quality and quantity of sperm. A fine needle is used to extract the healthy sperm best suited for fertilisation. The sperm are washed from the semen. If the quality of the sperm is poor, micro-manipulation techniques like ICSI may be recommended (see page 38).

STAGE 4: FERTILISATION
The sperm and egg are placed in a Petri dish for fertilisation to take place, as it would in the fallopian tube. If ICSI (see page 38) is used the sperm is injected directly into the egg using very fine instruments to assist fertilisation.

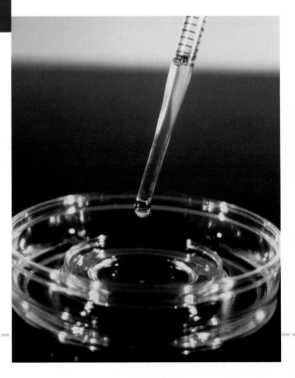

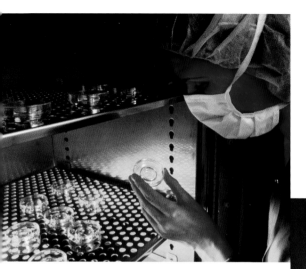

STAGE 5: MONITORING
The fertilised ova are placed in an incubator and are carefully watched. One or all of the eggs may be successfully fertilised. The fertilised cell is called an embryo. The embryologist will monitor the embryos for cell division (cleavage). The embryos will divide several times over the course of a few days.

Stage 6: Alternative procedures

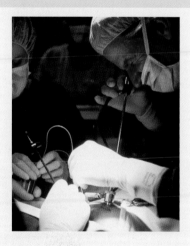

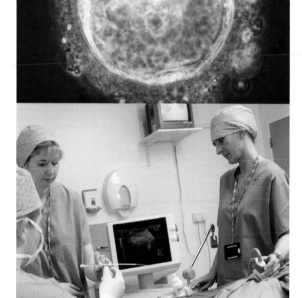

ZIFT (ZYGOTE INTRAFALLOPIAN TRANSFER)
The egg and sperm are fertilised outside the body and the resulting embryo is transferred to the fallopian tube.

GIFT (GAMETE INTRAFALLOPIAN TRANSFER)
The eggs and sperm are collected and transferred to the fallopian tube, so that fertilisation can take place within the body.

STAGE 6: EMBRYO TRANSFER
A maximum of two are selected to be placed back into the woman's body. The embryos that are not used may be frozen for future use. Using very fine instruments, the embryos are placed inside the uterus for implantation to take place.

Both partners will need a blood test to confirm they are not carriers of HIV, Hepatitis C or Hepatitis B. The clinic may offer a blood test on the day of your consultation or alternatively your doctor may be able to organise these tests for you and send the results to the clinic.

Other essential tests required are a rubella status, full blood count, and a day 1–3 hormone assessment for the woman. Many clinics may also test for the presence of anti phospholipid antibodies: an APLA test. The more information gained at this stage stands you in better stead later. Even if you have previously had IVF treatment and completed these blood tests during the last cycle, it is a requirement to have new tests every twelve months.

Fertility investigations

The clinic may require additional information about how your body and hormones work before starting treatment. The investigations may include monitoring a normal monthly cycle, assessing the internal health of your uterus and checking the functioning of your immune system.

Mid-cycle scan (cycle monitoring) Following the consultation, the doctor may wish to see how your natural hormones respond at the beginning, middle and end of your monthly cycle. Cycle monitoring usually involves a hormone profile blood test at the beginning of your period (days 1–3). A mid-cycle scan will usually be scheduled for a few days before your ovulation is due. The scan is performed by the doctor inserting an ultrasound probe into your vagina once your bladder is empty. The doctor is making an assessment of the lining of your womb and the activity of the ovaries at that time. Following the scan, a blood test will confirm your hormone levels at that stage of your cycle. You will then be asked to confirm when a surge in LH (luteinising hormone) has been detected. Ovulation predictor kits like Clearplan@ can be bought from most pharmacies. Once a positive result has been detected, call the clinic with the date; you may be required to have a further scan 5–6 days later. Further blood tests may be ordered to complete the picture. All this

information helps the doctor see how your body behaves at different stages of your natural cycle, and provides vital information on the best way to progress with IVF treatment.

Hysteroscopy On some occasions the doctor may require more information about you and your body and may wish to look internally at the health of your uterus.

A hysteroscopy is a procedure in which a small telescope-like instrument is inserted into the uterine cavity through the vagina (see page 79). Fluid is then used to distend the uterine cavity and abnormalities such as polyps, intrauterine fibroids and scar tissue can be seen.

Specific measurement of the uterine cavity can also be taken at this time. These measurements will assist your doctor in understanding the shape of your uterus, the way it is tilted and potentially the best place to position the embryo during embryo transfer. A hysteroscopy is a simple day-case procedure. Ideally, it is performed as close to the start date of your treatment cycle as possible.

Immune screening The study of immunology and its role in pregnancy and miscarriage is in its infancy. Many clinics are interested in assessing a couple's immunological status prior to embryo transfer to ensure there are no obvious reasons why the embryo may be rejected.

A profile of blood tests indicates the status of the immunological environment within a woman's reproductive system. The environment needs to be in optimum condition in order to allow successful implantation of an embryo in the uterus and for the resulting pregnancy to flourish. These blood tests tend to be costly as they are very specialised, may be sent overseas, and may take one to two weeks to process. The doctor will discuss with you the results and any implications.

Confirmation of treatment protocol

Once all the necessary information has been gathered, a treatment protocol will be discussed with you. Essentially this means the doctor will have decided whether to shut down your natural bodily systems before building up your hormone levels again or use your own hormones to kick-start the treatment. There are two types: a long protocol and a short protocol.

Long protocol Called a 'down regulation', this involves shutting down your natural hormones prior to ovulation stimulation. Typically, medication in the form of a nasal spray (Synarel) or a small daily injection will be given for a period of 10 to 14 days. The doctor will decide when you should start the medication, how much to take and at what time of day. It is important to remember to take the medication at the specified times, as the regularity of taking it say, every twelve hours, ensures the body 'shuts down' and regulates accordingly. Typically, medication is taken either seven days before your period starts (day 21) called 'luteal phase protocol' or on day two of your period, called 'follicular phase protocol'.

After 10 to 14 days on the medication, you will have a vaginal ultrasound scan to check that your ovaries and womb have successfully responded to the medication. A blood test may also be performed to measure the hormone levels at that time. The results will confirm if you are ready to start the stimulation drugs.

Short or 'flare' protocol This omits the down regulation phase and commences at the beginning of your menstrual cycle. All other aspects of the protocol are the same as a long protocol. Your doctor will know from all the fertility testing which protocol will suit you best. Short protocol tends to be recommended for women who have previously responded poorly to stimulation, older women and women with previously raised FSH levels. Following the day one hormone profile, which measures the FSH, LH, oestradiol and prolactin levels, you may be advised to have an ultrasound scan the following morning, when a final decision is made.

The fertility drugs

Now that your treatment has been confirmed, your doctor will prescribe a cocktail of fertility drugs and may tweak them over the course of the treatment. A woman's natural monthly cycle is completely stopped so that the fertility drugs can mimic the action of the hormones in a controlled manner. Normally a woman ovulates one egg per month. Fertility drugs are designed to work to stimulate the body to produce more than one egg a cycle. The mid-cycle monitoring has helped your doctor understand what happens naturally, so that fertility drugs can be taken appropriately. It is very unlikely that two women will take the same dosage of the same drugs for the entire IVF process.

The fertility drugs fall into the following categories:

Suppression drugs These are used to 'turn off' the natural secretion of FSH and LH during treatment and suppress ovulation until the follicles are mature. There are two types, GnRH (gonadotrophin-releasing hormone) agonists, which initially stimulate the release of FSH and LH from the pituitary. Taken over a sustained period they effectively 'turn off' the release of FSH and LH. Lupron and Synarel are common brand names. The second type is GnRH antagonists, which turn off the release of FSH and LH within several hours of an injection and have no initial stimulation effect. Cetrotide is a common brand name.

Stimulation drugs: HMG (Human Menopausal Gonadotrophin) is used to stimulate the development of multiple follicles and produce mature eggs. Some contain just FSH whereas other medications contain both FSH and LH. Your doctor will decide which is the most suitable for you. Common brand names include: Merional, Menogon, Menopure (containing FSH and LH), and Gonal F and Puregon (containing FSH alone).

Egg maturation After 10 days or more on stimulating drugs, the eggs within the follicles will be reaching maturity. An injection of HCG (human chorionic gonadotrophin) is taken to mimic the natural surge of LH (luteinising hormone) and leads to the final maturation of the eggs within the follicles. The injection is taken approximately 36 hours before egg collection. Common brands names are Ovitrelle and Pregnyl.

Raised FSH levels

In the event that the blood test on day 1–3 reveals raised FSH and/or oestradiol levels, you will be informed that treatment is not advisable in that cycle. The reason for this is that hormone levels indicate how well you will respond to the medications given to stimulate your ovaries. If the levels are raised, your ovaries are less likely to respond and produce good quality eggs. Clinics tend to vary on the levels with which they are happy, some preferring levels of FSH to be below 10. Research has shown that levels greater than 10 do not respond as well to fertility treatment and reduce the chance of a successful pregnancy. Details of what it means to have high FSH and oestradiol levels can be found on page 77.

Being told after all the testing that you cannot progress this month is devastating news. It seems you have put your life on hold, had numerous blood tests and scans and feel mentally ready to start; weeks have already passed since the initial consultation. I was unable to start treatment for five months due to high FSH levels every month. I was told monthly hormones could be erratic, especially in older women, and to be patient. It is better to wait for the one good month rather than risk taking all the fertility drugs, only to fail. Patience tends to be an attribute that infertile couples become accustomed to, I would not say it was a natural attribute, just one that develops during this process to have a baby. Be prepared, because when your FSH levels are good it will all happen very quickly!

Implantation and pregnancy After egg collection you may be prescribed additional medication to increase the chance of implantation and pregnancy. Progesterone is necessary because it prepares the uterine lining to receive a possible pregnancy, and is necessary to maintain pregnancy, should a pregnancy occur. Daily progesterone pessaries are recommended. Cyclogest is a common brand.

Additional medication: based on your medical history, your doctor may prescribe additional medication to encourage pregnancy and prevent miscarriage. For example, Ritodrine tablets help prevent muscle contractions occurring within the uterus; these contractions could potentially dislodge the embryo or prevent implantation. Heparin (Clexane) injections and aspirin are responsible for thinning the blood thereby increasing the blood flow to the uterus and preventing blood clotting. Evidence has shown a correlation between miscarriage and blood clots.

Ovarian stimulation

Now you are ready to start stimulating your ovaries in a controlled manner. Your doctor will prescribe the exact dosage of stimulation drugs each day at a specific time. The nurse will show you how to mix the drugs yourself and where to inject the needle. Stimulation drugs tend to be taken subcutaneously at a 45-degree angle in the skin of the stomach or in the thigh. At first, the prospect of injecting yourself with needles every day can be daunting. If you feel you cannot do it yourself, ask your partner or a member of your family to help you. To avoid bruising, insert the needle slowly into the skin at a 45-degree angle and withdraw slowly. Do not rub the site of injection afterwards. Arnica cream is quite good at reducing bruising. Ensure you are taking adequate vitamin C (500 mg) per day, as this not only will help with bruising but also, after egg collection, it will help to reduce any soreness or swelling in your uterus prior to embryo transfer.

Be prepared to visit the clinic often for blood tests and/or scans in the next 10–14 days. Clear your diary as much as possible. Try not to put yourself under pressure as the process of visiting the clinic, having blood tests and scans can be gruelling. Most couples fit in IVF treatment during their normal working day. Clinics tend to open early in the morning so blood tests can be done before the working day starts. Blood results are processed within hours so that your doctor can make an assessment of how you are responding that day. You may receive a phone call later in the day with an update on your oestradiol levels and any adjustments that need to be made to your dosage that night. I like to keep a daily record of my oestradiol levels rising as it helps me feel included in the process and I can see my body responding positively. I still feel in charge of my fertility even though a professional is helping me get pregnant!

After a few days, you will be into an established routine (see box).

It is highly recommended during the stimulation phase that you drink copious amounts of water. The doctor will usually recommend at least two litres of water and a half to one litre of milk to ensure you are well hydrated and minimise the risk of developing hyperstimulation. If your blood tests reveal your levels are rising too quickly or you have signs of overstimulation, this amount of fluid may be increased. This regimen should continue after your egg collection right up until the time of your pregnancy test. If at any stage you feel unwell, become bloated, experience nausea or vomiting, please let your doctor and his team know immediately. In addition, eating about 60 g of protein a day in the form of cheese, eggs, nuts and dairy products is recommended.

Egg collection

After 10-14 days of taking the stimulation drugs you will have a final scan to count the number of follicles, assess their size and determine if the lining of your womb is ready for implantation a few days later. Usually a measurement of between 7–10mm indicates the womb lining is ready. Some women may be ready after ten days; others may require stimulation until day 14. When you are ready you will be asked to take an evening injection of HCG (Human chronionic gonadotrophin) in preparation for the egg

A typical day on medication

Once you've embarked on fertility treatment an average day will be much like the following:

- early a.m.: Wake up and take any prescribed medication; visit the clinic for a blood test.

- midday: Receive phone call.

- afternoon: You may have to visit the clinic again for another blood test and/or scan, especially towards the final stages of ovarian stimulation (not all women).

- early evening: Take injection and take any other medication prescribed.

- night: Bed and a good night's sleep.

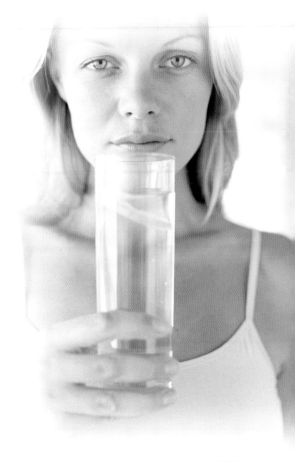

Micromanipulation techniques

After the egg and sperm have been collected, the embryologist may decide that he or she can increase the number of fertilised embryos by manipulating the egg and/or sperm, to assist fertilisation or implantation. These methods are called micromanipulation techniques and include ICSI, surgical aspiration of sperm and assisted hatching (AH).

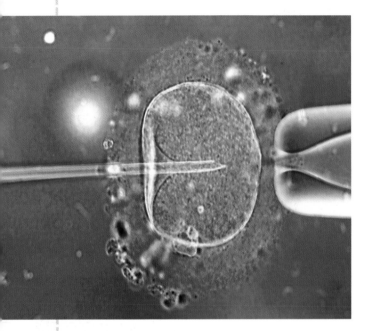

ICSI

Intracytoplasmic sperm injection has been hugely successful in improving a couple's chance of pregnancy if the man has sub-optimal sperm. In the majority of cases of male infertility, the sperm is not capable of penetrating the outer coating of the egg (zona pellucida) and so fertilisation is not possible. In recent years a number of techniques to facilitate breaking through the zona pellucida have been developed. The first human pregnancy after transferring embryos produced as a result of this technique occurred in 1988.

Microinjection of the sperm directly into the egg has been successful since 1991. Over 90 percent of couples treated by ICSI achieve fertilisation. The fertilisation rate per egg is about 60 percent.

Candidates for ICSI

After examining the sperm under a microscope the embryologist will decide on whether ICSI will enhance your chances. Typically ICSI is performed if:

- Previous treatment resulted in failure to fertilise or less than 30 percent of the eggs fertilised.

- The woman is a poor responder to ovarian stimulation, producing less than five eggs and less than 50 percent of the eggs fertilised.

- There are less than half a million progressive motile sperm in the preparation.

- The man has less than 10 percent morphologically normal sperm.

- There are high levels of anti-sperm antibodies present.

- Sperm has been collected from a surgical operation i.e. epididymal sperm aspiration (MESA PESA) or testicular sperm aspiration.

SURGICAL ASPIRATION OF SPERM

It is essential to collect sperm to fertilise the egg. One of the causes of male factor infertility is obstructive azoospermia in which no sperm can be found in the semen. This may be due to past infections damaging tissue, previous male sterilisation procedures (vasectomy) or congenital reasons. In such instances sperm can be aspirated surgically from the epididymis, the fine tubule of the testicle, in a procedure known as PESA (percutaneous epididymal sperm aspiration) or MESA (microsurgical epididymal sperm aspiration). Sperm may also be extracted directly from the testicular tissue by a procedure called TESE (testicular sperm aspiration). These techniques require a general anaesthetic and are performed on a day case basis.

As surgically aspirated sperm tend to be low in number and motility, ICSI is recommended, to increase the chance of fertilisation.

ASSISTED HATCHING (AH)

This is a technique used to improve the implantation of the embryos. The egg 'shell' (zona pellucida) is breached to allow the embryo to break free (hatch) and implant into the uterine lining. This technique may be helpful in women over 40 years of age. Special drugs (antibiotics and steroids) are required to be taken by the women undergoing this technique.

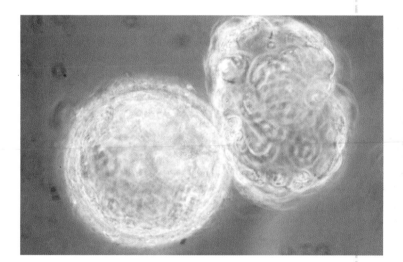

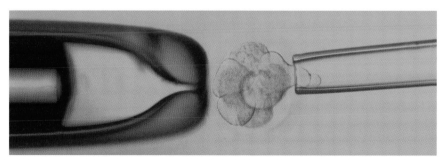

PGD (PRE-IMPLANTATION GENETIC DIAGNOSIS)

This is performed at some clinics to screen for inherited diseases. In PGD, one or two cells are removed from the developing embryo and tested for specific genetic diseases. Embryos that do not have the gene associated with the diseases are selected for transfer to the uterus. Recently, removing one or two cells from the embryo on day three to screen the embryo for the number of chromosomes it contains (pre-implantation genetic screening) has been suggested as a means of improving IVF results. Ask your doctor about this option.

Choose a treatment

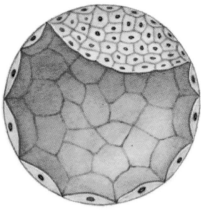

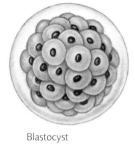

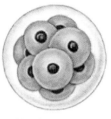

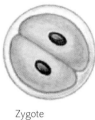

Zygote

Morula

Blastocyst

Blastocyst cross-section

THE DEVELOPING EMBRYO

Through a process of cell division known as mitosis, the ferilised ovum becomes a two-cell zygote, then continues to divide creating a morula, which is a cluster of solid cells, before turning into a 100-cell blastocyst.

collection 36 hours later. You will then take no more stimulatory drugs or down regulation drugs. If you have been taking other medication, you may be asked to stop taking it before egg collection and recommence afterwards.

Egg collection is performed under deep sedation anaesthesia administered by a consultant anaesthetist. It is essential that you do not eat or drink from midnight the day before until egg collection has been completed. The procedure usually takes between 20–30 minutes, is pain free and you are able to return home accompanied by your partner approximately three hours after sedation. The doctor will tell you immediately upon waking how many eggs have been collected.

While you are having your eggs collected, your partner is required to give a semen sample on the premises. Usually a private room is provided and the sample is collected in a small plastic container. The sample is then assessed for sperm quality, motility and abnormal forms by the embryology team.

Once the sperm has been prepared and immediately following egg collection, sperm is mixed with the eggs for fertilisation to occur.

In many cases, a micromanipulation technique such as ICSI (intracytoplasmic sperm injection) or AH (assisted hatching), (see pages 134–5) may be recommended at this stage to increase the chance of fertilisation.

Following egg collection, it is important to ready the uterus for the arrival of the embryos.

The doctor may prescribe progesterone pessaries (Cyclogest) to support their implantation.

Embryo monitoring

Embryos resulting from IVF, ICSI and AH are transferred between two to five days after egg collection. An embryologist will telephone you the morning following egg collection to tell you how many eggs have fertilised overnight. The embryos are monitored and examined on a daily basis to check for cell division (cleavage).

Each day the embryos may advance to the next stage of development i.e. from a two-cell embryo to a four-cell embryo. The embryologist is looking for a steady advancement in cell division and is trying to assess which are the best ones for embryo transfer.

The embryologist will call you with an update each day. The conversation may go something like this: "You have eight fertilised embryos, two of which are two cells, three are three cells and three are at the four-cell stage". The following day, the report may be "You have two three-cell embryos, four five-cell embryos and two eight-cell embryos, of which two are looking really good!" Based on the daily changes, the embryologist will decide when the ideal day for embryo transfer will be.

Embryo transfers take place typically on day two to three or five days after egg collection. At five days following egg collection, the embryos will be at the developmental stage known as blastocyst and therefore transfer on day five is

Difficulties and risks

There is always a downside and this section on IVF would not be complete without covering any difficulties that may be encountered during the treatment cycle and risks of having treatment.

- The IVF cycle may be abandoned if not enough follicles can be stimulated. This may occur in about 10 percent of cases.

- In less than one percent of cases, there may be a failure to retrieve any eggs from the follicles.

- Fertilisation may fail in some instances, but this has been quite low since the introduction of ICSI (intracytoplasmic sperm injection).

- Severe ovarian hyperstimulation (see pages 60–61) can develop. If the rare symptoms of nausea, vomiting, abdominal pain and distension develop at any time during treatment, the cycle may be abandoned.

- The chance of multiple pregnancy increases when more than one embryo is transferred. To some this is the desired outcome and the risks far outweigh the pluses. Twins tend to be born earlier and a woman carrying a twin pregnancy may need to spend weeks in bed or in hospital in an attempt to delay a premature delivery.

- Approximately 20–25 percent of all assisted reproduction pregnancies will miscarry. This is slightly higher than normally conceived pregnancies. The incidence of ectopic pregnancy following IVF is three percent of those who achieve pregnancy and is slightly higher (five percent) in those who conceive after GIFT (Gamete intrafallopian transfer), or ZIFT (Zygote intrafallopian transfer.

called a 'blastocyst transfer'. If a number of your embryos are healthy and developing successfully, your doctor may recommend you have a blastocyst transfer. Embryos tend to show a lot of differentiation between days three and five and on day three your doctor may be unable to decide which are the best two to transfer. A blastocyst transfer can increase the chances of pregnancy by up to 15 percent.

If there are remaining embryos suitable for freezing, the clinic will ask if you consent to freezing and storage, and an additional charge is levied. Consider it like paying for board and lodgings! A frozen embryo cycle is simpler, less expensive and less invasive that the initial IVF cycle, since the woman does not require ovarian stimulation or egg collection. The embryos may be frozen for several years. Not all embryos survive the freezing and thawing process and the live birth rate for frozen embryo cycles is lower than fresh cycles. That said, an estimated 15,000–20,000 babies in the UK have been born using frozen, thawed embryos.

Embryo transfer

Congratulations! You have waited many months and finally the day has come to place the embryos into your body. This can be quite an exciting time for a couple. Excitement, nervousness and anticipation are all common feelings at this time.

For this procedure, both partners can be present; in fact, it is usually recommended as it is such an important emotional moment in the IVF process.

The procedure is pain free. A soft, very fine catheter is passed though the cervix. Once this is in place, the embryos are transferred into the uterus with great precision. The procedure may take 20–30 minutes. You can leave whenever you feel comfortable to do so.

The doctor may prescribe additional medications to encourage blood flow to the uterus and to help implantation processes. It is still important to drink large amounts of water – two to three litres a day – as the stimulatory drugs are still circulating in your body. Drinking water will help flush them out.

The most important advice you will be given is to rest completely for two days, i.e. bed rest! I know it may sound excessive but there is a reason it is recommended. Implantation of embryos takes place between days 6-8 of their development. Following a two-, three- or five-day transfer, your body needs to be in a position to accept the embryos and encourage implantation processes to occur. By minimising your activities, blood is circulating to your uterus and any sudden movements are avoided. I have seen many women jump back into their working life the day after embryo transfer, only to question why they did not become pregnant. Would it have made a difference? For the sake of two days bed rest, I'm never willing to take that

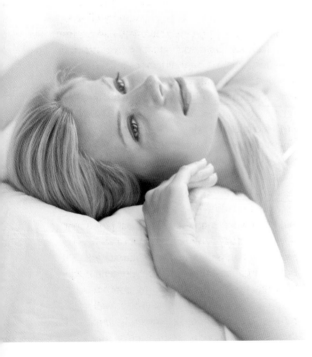

risk. I have always followed the clinic's advice to the letter so far, had a successful embryo transfer, and felt happy that I have done everything I needed to do to maximise my chance of conception.

Going home after embryo transfer is a great moment! You are happy in the knowledge that you have one or two little embryos inside and it is now up to your body to respond and encourage implantation and pregnancy. If you have been taking your vitamins and minerals for the last few months, your body will be in good reproductive health. Spend time visualising yourself with a baby. Give your embryos a name. Identify with them and, most importantly, relax. There is no point worrying at this stage, just enjoy every moment and reflect on what you have been through. You have come so far!

THE WAITING GAME – AM I PREGNANT?

Over the next two weeks, time will drag on forever. Each day following embryo transfer you will have a mixed bag of emotions. One day you may wake up feeling great and even feel pregnant, other days you will have doubts and feelings of negativity. To be honest, I have never found the ideal way to cope with this time. Despite reading numerous articles and listening to people's advice, I've always found it difficult.

I keep myself mentally busy yet physically inactive. I write copious lists of jobs to do around the house (and then give them to my husband!), update all our filing, sort out my clothes (by colour!), anything to distract me from thinking too much about the outcome. If I have moments when it all gets too emotional, I try to calm down, breathe deeply for 10–15 minutes and re-focus positively on how far I have come.

Two weeks seems like an eternity and most women will have been given a date by their clinics to have a pregnancy blood test. Most clinics prefer you to wait until day 14 and confirm it with a blood test at the clinic. The reason for this is to avoid any unnecessary false news. Over-the-counter pregnancy kits when taken early can produce a negative result, when a more sensitive blood test will show that you are actually pregnant. It is incredibly hard to resist buying one of these early pregnancy kits just to see if you are pregnant. Regardless of advice, most of us will not be able to resist the temptation of knowing at the soonest possible moment. Do what you need to do to keep yourself sane!

It's positive!

The two weeks have now passed and you have the results of your pregnancy test. If the results are positive, huge congratulations to you both! You are pregnant! Cherish this moment. The difficult part is over and you now have nine months ahead of you to enjoy being pregnant and preparing yourself for parenthood. Now that you are pregnant the clinic may adjust the medications you have been taking to ensure your body is healthy and help to prevent miscarriage.

It is only natural now that you are pregnant to have thoughts and fears of losing the baby. The next twelve weeks are an essential time for the development of your baby. Keep visualising yourself with a baby. Surround yourself with positive people and positive thoughts. Many women having undergone the IVF process are so happy to be pregnant, the positive wave of emotions carries them through the difficult times.

Keep taking your pre-conception vitamins and minerals – especially folic acid – for the next three months.

It's negative ...

If the result of your pregnancy test is negative, you and your partner will be devastated. The tears and words of sympathy from family and friends cannot express how you are feeling inside. Crushed, empty, lost and sorry for yourselves. It feels like someone has ripped out your heart and you cannot see how you could ever recover from this. The IVF process has been incredibly demanding of your time, emotions and strength. And now you have been told you are not pregnant! There is no easy way to move on from this.

Take one day at a time. If close family and friends have been aware of you having IVF, now is the time to call upon their support. You may

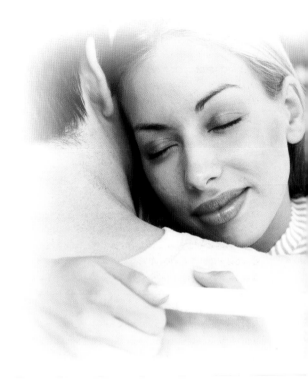

be surprised at how sympathetic and understanding they are. Or you can use the counselling services offered by fertility clinics. Counselling is a process where you can explore your feelings about your situation in a safe and accepting environment. It is non-judgmental and strictly confidential. When treatment is unsuccessful or no longer appropriate, the counsellor can help in allowing you to express your feelings and come to terms with your disappointment. In this way potential damage to your relationship can be minimised or prevented.

There is no point blaming each other for the lack of success. Now is the time to come together and unite to deal with the situation. Men and women do deal with disappointment in different ways and for the sake of saving a marriage, counselling may be ideal for you both. It may be a way of helping you deal with your emotions without worrying about how your partner may react. Fertility counsellors have a high level of expertise and training in the field of infertility.

VARIATIONS OF IVF

IVF is the by far the most popular method of assisted conception. Slight variations on the IVF process exist and may be recommended depending on a couple's circumstances.

GIFT

In Gamete Intrafallopian Transfer, the fertility drugs protocols are identical to IVF, the main difference being in the retrieval and transfer procedures. The eggs are collected laparoscopically and the gametes (egg and sperm) are transferred to the woman's fallopian tubes rather than her uterus. GIFT is only an option for women who have normal fallopian tubes. Some couples may consider GIFT for religious reasons because eggs are not fertilised outside the body.

ZIFT

Zygote Intrafallopian Transfer differs from GIFT in that fertilisation takes place outside the woman's body although, again, the fertilised egg is transferred to the fallopian tube rather than the uterus.

SUSAN'S STORY

The worst part of it all is the waiting ... And the fact that there is nothing you can do, except wait. To begin with we were waiting for each period to come and wishing it wouldn't, then we were waiting to get the appointment, then to start the tests, which were inconclusive, then there was waiting for the IVF clinic appointment, timing the first cycle, waiting within each cycle and then the long two weeks after implantation, which ended in acute disappointment.

After the first four IVF cycles each producing fewer eggs (the final one being downgraded to insemination because I only produced two eggs), it became apparent that this was not going to work. Although a high proportion of the eggs successfully fertilised – and, for a short while, I was actually pregnant – we were both aware that to continue along the same lines would be obsessive behaviour. We discussed the options with the consultant who recommended trying egg donation at a clinic where this method was a specialty. This, of course, came with more waiting – first for the initial appointment and then for a donor; the waiting list for an anonymous donor was at least 12 months.

We were overwhelmed by the generosity of friends and relatives who offered to act as donors, unfortunately most were 'too old'. (Imagine having to say, "Thank you but you are too old" to someone who is offering the most amazing gift possible.) Two people were potential donors and to choose between them was impossible without help from the counsellor attached to the IVF clinic. Twelve months after we began the treatment our wonderful baby boy was born – people think nine months is a long wait. Just to rub it in, Jack was as overdue as possible – keeping us waiting to the end.

Many people write about how IVF destroyed their marriage. Throughout the years of frustration, we have never lost sight of the fact that this is about 'us' and our relationship is stronger as a result. We focused on ensuring that we did not become obsessive and recognised that the frustration and disappointment was shared. Our friends and family also provided wonderful support (not to mention other kids to play with). It certainly wasn't easy, especially when we lost the first pregnancy at 12 weeks, but we now have a beautiful little boy – and that is what it was all about.

Sperm/egg and embryo donation

IVF may be done with a couple's own eggs and sperm or with donor eggs, sperm or embryos. A couple may choose this route if there is a problem with their own sperm or eggs or if they have a genetic disease that could be passed on to a baby. In the UK, about 1,570 babies a year are born using donated sperm, egg or embryos.

Sperm donation

This is an option for men who have poor quality and/or quantity of sperm or who have had a vasectomy. Single women and lesbian couples wishing to have a baby also use donated sperm to conceive a baby. The process involves using a very fine tube to deposit sperm at the neck of the womb or into the womb at a time that coincides with the natural release of an egg. The sperm is usually supplied by an anonymous donor who has undergone extensive medical and genetic screening. Donors are between 18 and 45 years old, have been screened for infections such as AIDS, hepatitis and any genetic illnesses.

In April 2005, the legal position regarding donor anonymity changed. Children from donations now have access to information about their genetic origins. This includes the donor's name, latest known address, date of birth, town and district of birth and appearance. On reaching 18, anyone born from a donation can apply to the HFEA to receive information about the donor.

According to the latest HFEA figures, with each attempt, donor inseminated women under 30 years old have a 13.5 percent chance of having a baby. At 35–39 years of age, this drops to 9 percent and for the over 40s is 2.5 percent.

Egg donation

This is suitable for women who are unable to produce their own eggs. The most common reasons women choose egg donation is they suffer from premature ovarian failure (early menopause), they have no ovaries or their ovaries have been removed, an illness such as cancer has caused infertility or several attempts

at IVF have been unsuccessful. In the UK, 5,500 babies have been born following egg donation since 1991.

It is a three-way process, involving a donor, the recipient woman and a man. The donor must undergo ovarian stimulation and egg collection. During this time, the recipient takes hormones to prepare her uterus for the arrival of the fertilised egg. The male has provided a sperm sample, which has been washed and prepared. If the sperm are of poor quality or motility, ICSI may be offered at this stage to increase the chance of fertilisation. The best embryos are selected and transferred into the recipient woman for implantation to occur and to carry the pregnancy to full term.

The success rates for egg donation are higher than traditional IVF as most donors tend to be young, healthy females aged under 36 years. The success rates are 25–40 percent for each attempt.

Embryo donation

If both the man and woman are unable to use their own sperm or eggs, embryo donation may be the ideal option. Donated embryos tend to be from IVF couples who have decided to donate their spare embryos to help other infertile couples have a baby. The recipient woman receives the embryo in the same way as one undergoing frozen embryo transfer.

Diary of an IVF cycle

AUGUST

31st

Wednesday Today is day two of my period and after four months of hormone testing I think we have found the lowest FSH levels yet and can start treatment this month. The clinic called to confirm we can go ahead and need to see me tomorrow for an internal ultrasound exam.

SEPTEMBER

1st

Thursday Had lots of positive comments during my scan; ovaries and womb look healthy so we are progressing to the next stage. They decided that the best protocol for me is a luteal down regulation so I start the nasal spray today. One spray in both nostrils twice a day! I'll do this for six days and have another scan to see if I have shut down.

7th

Wednesday Bad news! Not only have I been feeling moody and emotional from the spray in the last week but the scan showed I haven't completely shut down. My ovaries started to develop an egg naturally. In order to progress we need to wait until the next period! I'm gutted! Been given some tablets to help accelerate this and should get it within 7–10 days.

23rd

Friday Period came today and I'm miles away from the clinic at a friend's wedding. Called the clinic and they can do a day 3

assessment so I will get up early on Sunday and hotfoot it to the clinic for a blood test.

25th

Sunday (day 1) Hooray; we can start treatment! Need to get myself organised as the clinic will want to see me every day for the next two weeks. I have chosen a clinic 200 miles away, must find accommodation immediately. Started my injections today. It's a bit nerve wracking doing the first one. Is it the right dose? Will it hurt? Simon helped me with the first one into my abdomen, it was slow but painless thankfully!

26th

Monday (day 2) Checked into a hotel first thing and rushed over to the clinic for my first blood test to see how I responded to last night's injection. By 4 p.m. the clinic called with my instructions on the next dosage. Injection tonight easier. Finding it hard to increase my water intake – up to about 3 litres a day and it's still not enough!

27th

Tuesday (day 3) Got to the blood test by 9 a.m. Felt a bit dizzy afterwards as they took six vials of blood today – one to measure my oestradiol daily levels, all the others for an immune test. Apparently, if a woman has a high number of natural 'killer' cells, she may reject the developing embryo early on in pregnancy. This test will show if I need to take any precautions. Call at 5 p.m. confirmed tonight's dosage.

28th

Wednesday (day 4) Feeling tired today – had a sleep at lunchtime after my daily blood test. Eating lots of protein snacks throughout the day. My dosage has been reduced for the last two days as my blood tests show my oestradiol levels are high and I have responded well to the drugs.

29th

Thursday (day 5) Had a blood test twice today. Each time you see some familiar faces at the clinic. Most sit in silence but you do get the occasional person who is happy to talk and swap stories. How many times have you had IVF? What stage are you at? What day of stimulation? What drugs are you taking? After a while you can tell who is at what stage by the size of the water bottle: the larger the bottle, the closer the woman is to egg collection as she probably has increased her quantity up to 4 litres like me! The waiting room offers a great opportunity to talk to people who can identify with your situation. I met a woman who was on her sixth attempt, another who successfully had an IVF baby and wanted child number two! By sharing, you feel informed, confident and not alone; these are real women going through it with you at the same time!

30th

Friday (day 6) Scan at 7:30 a.m. today to see how the follicles are developing. There were already 30 women in the waiting room at that time! My womb lining is thickening nicely and I have follicles on both ovaries but must drink even more fluids! Excited that I've now seen the follicles and potential eggs, I feel my body is working well. One of those follicles has the egg that will fertilise and create a beautiful baby. From now on, I'm with them every step of the way. It's so amazing! How can you explain to your son or daughter that you have seen them as the tiniest of cells?

OCTOBER

1st

Saturday (day 7) Received a call mid-morning after my blood test to ask if I could come back again for another test a few hours later. My oestradiol level has shot up from 3990 to 5927 overnight. It has been doubling almost every day – 57, 225, 858, 1591, 3429 – which is good. I am quite bloated, however, and have resorted to my good old drawstring trousers! I am told not to take any drugs that evening and come for another test the next morning.

2nd

Sunday (day 8) The clinic is so busy at the weekends. I cannot get over how dedicated the staff are and how much time they spend helping couples get pregnant. It seems they operate every day and never fail to call each night. Oestradiol levels are still rising and I am told not to take any drugs that night either. This is a relief to me as I feel like I'm going to pop! Not all women are sensitive to the drugs and we all react differently.

143

3rd

Monday (day 9) Struggled to get up this morning; had a bad night's sleep, very uncomfortable. Had blood test at 7:30 a.m. Drank 2.5 litres of water by 11 a.m. and ate lots of protein this morning. Despite not having drugs for two days, my oestradiol levels are now cruising at a swift 13,533!

4th

Tuesday (day 10) Feeling better and excited about having a scan this afternoon to see how many follicles have developed and if I am ready for my 'trigger' injection. Feel like I'm getting close now! After the scan, it was decided I needed one more day to ripen and thicken my endometrium, which is currently 7.9 mm.

5th

Wednesday (day 11) The morning blood test showed my oestradiol levels dropped right off – down to 8,331. I was told immediately to take a small dose of drugs and come back later to see if it did the trick! Sure enough, back to 14,000 and I'm ready for the trigger injection at 8:30 tonight! This means egg collection will be 8:30 Friday morning! I'm so excited and nervous! It means I get a day off from blood tests and scans tomorrow and maybe even can sleep in!

7th

Friday (day 13) Egg collection day. Up and out bright and early. There are seven other women there for egg collection as well. We all look slightly anxious, clutching our partners' hands. Within minutes of lying on the operating table, the

anaesthetic takes hold. I wake up with a dry throat, slightly drowsy and a little sore, which is to be expected. I am told they collected a lot of eggs – 26. I knew I felt like I was going to pop! Simon did his bit in a room upstairs and within a few hours we go home pleased that we have got this far. We have been told Simon's sperm is good for fertilisation so we do not need ICSI and they will call tomorrow with the results!

8th

Saturday (day 14) The embryologist called to say 15 eggs fertilised and they are doing well. We are over the moon. That's twice as many as last time and we are both two years older. At 39 I was always worried about my egg quality but the feedback lifts our spirits and now we wait to see how they progress.

9th

Sunday (day 15) The embryos are two days old now and we have a number of 2-to-5-cell embryos. I really look forward to the embryologist's calls – it's a report on how our babies are doing. They are looking at which ones are the best to put back in. We are told it is unlikely we will have a day 3 transfer tomorrow as there are so many to choose from. As the days progress, the embryos start differentiating themselves – it's like survival of the fittest!

10th

Monday (day 16) Nine embryos have progressed to eight cells today and one embryo is now a 10 cell. The embryologist positively reassures us of the good news and says he will now wait until day 5 to see if any embryos develop into blastocysts. A lot of changes happen over the next 24 hours and two clear winners should be identified. We are very happy; last time we had a day 3 transfer, as most of the embryos only survived the first few days, now they can't decide! Blastocyst transfers tend to have higher success rates as well so we are keen to take his advice.

12th **Wednesday (day 18)** Embryo transfer day. The embryos are five days old. The call in the morning said the clinic would like a few more hours to see what may happen. Simon and I have been at home for the last four days and it will take us 3–4 hours to drive to the clinic if we go ahead. The embryologist calls at 1p.m. – he would like to do it today. Two have divided again and look great! We jump in the car excited that we are finally putting them back. Despite being the last couple in the clinic, the embryo is successfully transferred under very calm, serene surroundings. I do feel at peace and very happy it has all worked out so far. Back home for two days' bed rest and sleep!

One week later I'm going insane! One minute I think I'm pregnant and my breasts feel tender, the next I'm in floods of tears worrying what I'll do if I'm not pregnant! I'm due to have my beta HCG blood test on Friday … two more days to go! Have to do it, have to buy an early pregnancy kit and find out if I'm pregnant.

Later that day Did the pregnancy test and a faint line came up! Does that mean I'm pregnant? It's quite faint but the box says the line will only show if it has detected the human growth hormone so … I must be right?? Persuade myself that I am but will not celebrate until I have the blood test results. Simon would prefer to wait for the conclusive results before celebrating.

Two days later Blood test results show that I am pregnant! We are over the moon, can't stop smiling! Told close family the good news. Now I just need to take it easy for the next eight weeks. Once we are over the 12-week hurdle, we can share the news with all our friends!

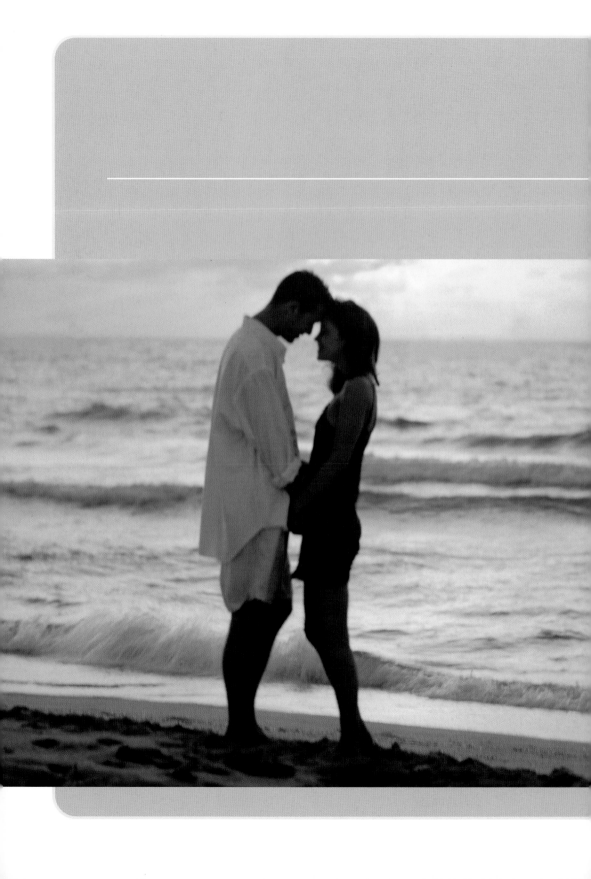

Emotional issues

As you continue to try for a baby you will experience many different emotional states. Understanding what they are and how to cope when they arise is key to maintaining your sanity and enjoying a happy relationship.

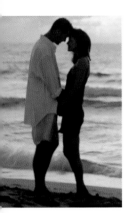

Infertility arouses an emotional side of you that you may not have experienced before. You will experience many ups and downs trying to fulfill your dream of having a baby. No two couples react the same way. Words used to describe the emotional experience include guilt, frustration, impatience, desperation, longing, anxiousness, embarrassment, failure, disappointment, anger, unfairness, heartache, grief, hope, anticipation, encouragement and excitement. All these emotions can be felt over a short period of time or last for years.

The first disappointment is the realisation that after months of trying for a baby you are not pregnant and that you and your partner may be infertile. Many couples find it hard to digest this news and their relationship becomes strained.

Next, you bare your soul to the doctors while they investigate what may be the cause of your infertility. This can be extremely imposing mentally and physically for both partners. Suddenly, every minute detail of your medical and sexual history is scrutinised, leaving no stone unturned! Physically you will be prodded and poked and any feeling of embarrassment soon dissipates after the third or fourth time.

You will emerge from fertility testing feeling relieved, anxious yet excited as the cause of infertility may be found so you can progress with treatment. Starting a treatment brings a wave of optimism, hope and anticipation that you will get pregnant. As the process continues this turns into fear; fear that it may not work and if it doesn't what will you do next? What else can you try? Then you experience the ultimate emotion, failure. The treatment has not worked and you are not pregnant and you are heartbroken. Men and women were meant to procreate but why not us? What have we done to deserve this? Why is it so easy for some people? The questions buzz around your head incessantly, driving you mad! Suddenly it seems that there are babies and pushchairs everywhere. At this time it is important to have the right emotional support to prevent you sliding into a depression.

So what can you do to help you cope?

Your relationship

It is important that you embark on this journey of having a baby together with a solid relationship. Infertility is such a personal issue that most couples tend not to share the news with anyone else initially. In some respects this is a good approach as it helps the couple come to terms with the issues themselves before being questioned by family and friends. It is important to be open with each other about how you feel and not hide your innermost thoughts. Keep yourself grounded by reminding yourself that you are a couple who fell in love years ago and are still in love. You can get through this together by talking about it and remembering how much fun you had before the baby pressures arrived. Revisit those feelings; take time to pamper each other, go out for meals and try to forget about the stress of having a baby for a while. Your relationship will invariably become stronger and your world will not solely revolve around having a baby.

If you find that you are arguing a lot, it may be time to share the news with family and friends so you can get the additional support you need. There is no point going round in circles, blaming each other and avoiding the issue. Confide in someone you can trust, someone else on whom you can vent your anger. Your partner is probably angry as well and when you come together, the fireworks will not help either of you to move on.

See the funny side Yes, believe it or not there is a funny side to infertility. You will have moments when you and your partner are in stitches laughing about a situation. He may be rushing home at lunchtime because he receives a call that you are 'ripe and ready'. You may be injecting your fertility drugs in the back of a car at a friend's wedding and get caught with your dress hitched up! After having sex you may bump into a friend going to the clinic for your post coital exam wondering why your legs are crossed. For your first ultrasound exam, you may get carried away and strip off all your clothes. You may take to having sex when it's a full moon because you have read it is important to be in tune with Mother Nature. When you are feeling down, reflect on some of the funny things that have happened and remember you are not alone. There are one in five couples also going through the same feelings and emotions as you are and trying to figure out a way forward.

Support groups

Confiding in family and/or friends can be very beneficial in dealing with your emotions if you are happy to share the information with familiar people. Many couples enjoy the anonymity of counselling and support groups as they feel they can be more honest about their true feelings. There are several support groups specifically set up to help infertile couples and most fertility clinics offer a counselling service. Phone a few and find the right one for you. You may not succeed the first time, but do not give up. Once you identify with someone, you will find it easier to talk.

Internet chat rooms are becoming increasingly popular, as you can be even more anonymous since you don't have to be physically present to get advice and feedback. It is easy to find a group of people who are in the same situation as you. Most chat rooms are divided into sub-groups; for example, there are chat rooms for women to discuss their IVF treatments, other rooms to discuss how you are feeling after a pregnancy test. Again, visit a few different sites

and sections until you find one that makes you feel comfortable. The main benefit of Internet chat rooms is the immediacy of the feedback; it's great for an instant pick-me-up. Unlike counselling, you do not have to wait for an appointment for a few days' time; people respond usually within the day.

Details on support groups and Internet sites can be found at the back of the book.

Financial help

Fertility treatment not only has emotional consequences but also financial consequences. Most couples have the added burden of finding a way to pay for their fertility treatment. Common methods include paying by credit card, borrowing from family, selling a car, re-mortgaging the house, and I've even heard of people downsizing their homes to pay for treatment. All this is an additional stress you do not need at such a difficult time. Try and avoid putting too much pressure on yourself by setting a budget and timescale. It is so easy to get carried away with having fertility treatment until it works. Also, sort out the finances before treatment starts so you can focus all your positive thoughts on the forthcoming treatment and getting pregnant.

Simon and I have had six IVF attempts over the last seven years, which have taken their toll emotionally, physically and financially. We have had to be creative with our finances and make sure we both agree on how we will raise and spend the money. Sacrifices have been made, sometimes reluctantly! Once you have a glimmer of hope of having a baby, you will find ways to fund the treatment until one day you decide enough is enough and you cannot afford to do this anymore. If you are not careful, treatment, especially numerous IVF attempts, can run into tens of thousands of pounds over the years. We have never added it up but one woman I met has spent almost £40,000 so far! Try not to let the financial side of infertility run away from you, if you can!

LOUISE'S STORY

I was referred to the hospital by my doctor as we had been trying for a baby for three years without success. My periods were extremely irregular so it was impossible to guess my 'fertile time'. The doctor I saw in the clinic examined my abdomen. Almost immediately she started smiling and told me she thought I was pregnant and asked me to produce a urine sample for a pregnancy test. The results took three minutes and we had to sit back in the waiting room. The minutes dragged by as we stared in disbelief at each other. I was so excited at the thought of possibly being pregnant after all this time. Eventually a nurse walked through the waiting room and just shook her head at us as she passed us. We were both very disappointed, but, soon after, all I could think was – if it wasn't a baby she had felt, what was it? The mass the doctor felt was attached to my ovary and I would have to have it removed. Never mind, I thought, you only need one ovary to get pregnant. Soon it became apparent that I had large cysts on both ovaries. All I remember was going to the toilet where I cried and cried with my poor husband left outside, unable to come to my aid. Why had I never considered the possibility that it would be on both ovaries?

The operation confirmed that the cysts were 'chocolate cysts' resulting from endometriosis that I had apparently been suffering from for years. I also had to have half of one ovary and two thirds of the other removed. The cysts were 8- and 10 cm in diameter and the consultant said it was rare to see a case so advanced. Endometriosis is usually a very painful condition and this is primarily how it is first diagnosed. I had always had period pain but had never had pain in between periods so that's how it went undetected for so long.

In addition to this, a dye test revealed that one fallopian tube was completely blocked and that the other side was almost completely blocked. This, I was told, was a result of scar tissue and adhesions from the operation. My only option for having a baby was IVF. The three-year waiting list on the NHS seemed too long. My husband is considerably older than me and armed with our savings and money from my mum, we embarked on our first attempt.

I am 28 years old and healthy and my chances of success were high I was told. We told the world what we were doing and, after so much recent heartache, were happy and positive about the IVF. I endured all the injections to the point where I felt like a pincushion, yet we still managed to find some humour in the process. The injections had to be done at the same time each day; one night we found ourselves in the car park of a hotel in the midst of my cousin's wedding reception, with my dress hitched up and my husband helping me with the injection. When someone walked past the car, heaven knows what they thought we were doing, but we did laugh about it afterwards.

Then there was a second course of IVF – more drugs, more hormones, more injections. During this treatment we only told very close family and no one else. I managed to arrange all the hospital appointments before work and so no one there knew either. During this cycle we were told that there was a problem with my husband's sperm as well – no problem with the count, but the motility was an issue and they recommended ICSI. This treatment also failed. As if turning 30 wasn't enough to be depressed about, the IVF failed on my 30th birthday and I was devastated.

Treatment number three was less invasive as we replaced the thawed embryos. It was the same emotional roller coaster, but not as much to be done physically. Unfortunately this treatment also failed, and at this point our clinic closed. We were faced with the further problem of finding a new clinic to continue the process.

We started afresh with treatment number four. Following another course of ICSI, I had two embryos replaced and went home with hope in my heart and everything crossed (literally!). This treatment also failed in December. Over Christmas, while I was still in the depths of depression, I found out my cousin was pregnant. I can't explain how or why I reacted the way I did, but I sunk to the lowest I had ever been. While growing up, my brother and I were very close to my two cousins and we used to discuss things, like who would get married first and who would have a baby first – it was everyone's opinion that I would be the one to do both first. I had managed the marriage part, but I think that's why I was so upset about the baby part.

Onwards and upwards though. We had embryos in the freezer from the fourth treatment, so in March we had treatment number five – another frozen transfer. By now I had decided that if the fresh cycle didn't work, then the frozen transfer was really a waste of time and I viewed it almost as something I had to do to get to the next fresh cycle, so this was the one I approached with the best mental attitude – in other words, the least stress. After two weeks I still hadn't bled, so I attended my appointment for the pregnancy test. I told the nurse that I felt as though I was going to start my period imminently and had been having mild period pains and so wasn't very hopeful. She smiled and told me not to worry yet. Even so, when I phoned up for the results that afternoon and was told that I was pregnant, I was dumbfounded and totally overjoyed!

Ten days later though, I bled very heavily and lost two big clots – I was convinced they were my embryos and was once again inconsolable. We went to the clinic the next day where we had a scan, and there it was – a heartbeat. I cannot even begin to describe the happiness or the relief we felt at that moment.

I carried on bleeding lightly for the next few weeks, but everything was still fine and after the morning sickness tapered off at about 17 weeks, I sailed through the pregnancy and enjoyed every second of it – in fact my friends think I mourned it when I was no longer pregnant.

On 10 December 2000 I gave birth to my son. The feeling is amazing and I have to admit that I am crying now, remembering it. He is beautiful and perfect and I love motherhood. He was born four months after my cousin's baby, also a boy, and they get on brilliantly – so everything really does happen for a reason!

THE MAN'S PERSPECTIVE

So what does the man in this experience make of it all? Well that's a difficult one! At the time my wife, Marina, was diagnosed with an inability to conceive naturally, I was at a point in my life where I couldn't really confess to a great longing to have a child at that time. Sure, I always wanted a family some day, but I was only 30 years old and it seemed a while away in my mind. This is, of course, until you are told that as a couple you may have difficulty in conceiving. Then, everything changes; even if you're not completely 'ready', you throw yourself positively into what may be a long and difficult journey.

I used to be medically naïve. Luckily, I have always been in good health, so before undergoing infertility treatment, doctors and I rarely crossed paths. When we began, I sat in front of a fertility expert who told me that in his professional opinion, Marina and I were part of the 25 percent of couples with unexplained infertility. I thought to myself, 'Am I really paying you to tell me you don't know what is wrong with us, because that is what you are saying, isn't it?' I was hoping for a more definitive message and all I felt was frustration and anger.

We became very persistent and wanted to know how we could improve our situation. Further tests revealed Marina had problems, which could only be overcome with intervention. This was a relief but I can honestly say I never blamed her as it had always been a case of 'we are in this together'. I adopted a fully supportive role and, to a certain degree, that is all a man can do, as the majority of treatments focus on the female. Watching your partner endure treatment can be difficult; you want to help more and share the burdens, but you can't.

After many years of trying naturally we turned to IVF with great hopes. This is where it all went horribly wrong for me as the first attempt failed and on the second attempt, Marina ended up in intensive care. I certainly questioned what we were doing. Was I prepared to lose the life of the closest person to me in the hope of having a baby? The simple answer was 'No!'

This was a big eye-opener to me; I had lost confidence in the IVF process. There had to be a better way. I am more than a little angry when I reflect back to this time. The difference between the clinic where we found success and the one that nearly cost my wife's life is like chalk and cheese. My advice to anyone is do your research, ask questions, and dig deeper than the literature. IVF is a developing science; even the experts are learning all the time about how to improve their success rates.

As a couple, be honest at all times with how you feel about what you're embarking on, and if you feel uncomfortable about it, say so! Trying for a baby is difficult and will drain you emotionally and physically. Address the financial issues; don't try and cope as you go along. Be supportive of each other, talk things through and have an endgame in sight, however unthinkable. You have to draw a line somewhere! But, most importantly, throughout your whole journey remain positive, stay focused on what you are trying to achieve – 'the big picture' – and take care of each other!

When enough is enough

When to stop trying for a baby is probably one of the hardest decisions a couple has to make. The most common reasons couples stop trying are physical, emotional and financial.

A woman may stop because she is physically unable to have any more treatment, the treatment has failed too many times, and the doctors do not know what else to suggest; or she is too old and does not have any eggs left.

A couple may decide that their relationship can't take the strain of infertility any more and want to draw a line under the experience, get their lives back to normal and have some fun!

Finally, you simply cannot afford to keep trying any longer as the money has run out and you cannot raise any more.

Some couples take years to decide they've had enough while others wake up one day and decide they want to get their life back to normal straightaway. Only you will know when you are ready to give up trying and move on.

Making this decision can bring a feeling of relief and freedom to you. No longer are you a slave to your monthly menstrual cycle; you can start to enjoy sex again at other times of the month besides ovulation. You can eat and drink what you like without feeling guilty and you can treat yourself to a nice holiday. You feel like you have been stuck in an infertility time warp and now you can move forward with your life.

When a couple reaches this point they may also be faced with another decision. Should they accept their life is one without a biological child of their own or look at other options for parenthood, such as adoption or surrogacy?

Other options for parenthood

Surrogacy and adoption may be considered by couples who are at the end of the road in their efforts to have a child. In the UK surrogacy appears to be an easier option than adoption. Both options have brought happiness to thousands of people, and if you are considering one of these options it is worth contacting the specialist agencies that deal with them.

Suitable for adoption?

Most agencies might not let you adopt if you:

- Are unmarried. Agencies prefer single women or married couples.
- Have not completed any fertility treatment six months prior to applying.
- Have a child that is less than two years older than the considered adopted child; most agencies prefer a larger age gap.
- Don't have enough physical space in your accommodation to provide for the child.
- Have a criminal conviction.
- Haven't been with your partner very long.
- Are in the process of moving house. Most agencies may suggest you delay until you are settled in your new home.
- Have recently suffered a death of a child in your family.
- Are under 21 years old.
- Have a history of mental illness.
- Are not a UK resident.

Surrogacy This is when another woman carries and gives birth to a baby for you. There are two types of surrogacy – straight and host surrogacy.

In *straight surrogacy*, the surrogate uses her own egg and fertilises it with the intended father's sperm. This is done by artificial insemination using a syringe. The baby will have the surrogate mother's genes and the male partner's genes. It is usually arranged privately and fertility clinics may assist if you wish to use their services for the intrauterine insemination.

In *host surrogacy*, the male partner's sperm fertilises the female partner's egg and the embryo is implanted into the womb of the surrogate by IVF. In this situation, the baby is genetically the couple's child and is unrelated to the surrogate.

If donated eggs are used to fertilise the sperm, the egg donor is the genetic mother; the surrogate carries the baby and is unrelated to the baby. For this the specialist services of an IVF clinic are required. Details of clinics providing this service can be found at the www.surrogacy.org.uk website.

Finding a surrogate can be difficult as they are not able to advertise their services. A friend or family member may offer to be a surrogate and organisations like COTS (Childlessness Overcome Through Surrogacy) may be able to point you in the right direction. Essentially, the surrogate needs to be a woman who is healthy, free of any congenital problems, can carry a baby to full term and is someone you can trust. You may worry that the surrogate may change her mind, which she is legally able to do even if the baby is not genetically related to her. This situation seems uncommon, but you should research the legal issues around surrogacy so you are fully aware of what it involves.

Adoption There are approximately 5,000 children adopted each year in the UK. Loving families care for these children as if they were their own children. Of the children adopted, 60 percent are between the ages of one and four years old, with only five percent being under one year old. Twenty-nine percent are aged between five and nine years old and only five percent are between 10 and 15. Many couples wish to adopt a young baby so they can bring up the baby from an early age as their own. It seems that children less than one year old are not often available and are usually only matched to couples aged between 26 and 35. If you are older and wishing to adopt, you may need to consider adopting an older child.

The adoption process is very thorough and as a result takes time. It is important that you as prospective parents attend adoption group sessions, which inform you of what to expect. You will be assessed by the agency; home visits may be arranged and references will be collected from your GP and other professionals. All this background is an essential part of matching you with the future 'right' child. Once

you have been approved as adopters, your agency will endeavour to find a suitable child for you. Recently, the government set up the National Adoption Register to make approved adopters available to social workers who work in other areas to help improve adoption rates.

Guidelines have been set out to help couples assess whether they would be eligible to become adoptive parents. Most agencies welcome couples that are heterosexual, gay or lesbian, are financially secure, employed, self-employed or unemployed, in good health and have a stable relationship.

When you adopt a child you become the child's legal parent and he or she will usually take your surname. The child will also inherit from you just as if he or she was born to you. Upon the granting of an adoption order, the child's natural parents will no longer have any rights or responsibilities towards the child. It is important that you are aware of the legal issues around adoption: www.adoption.org.uk has detailed information about adoption and its implications.

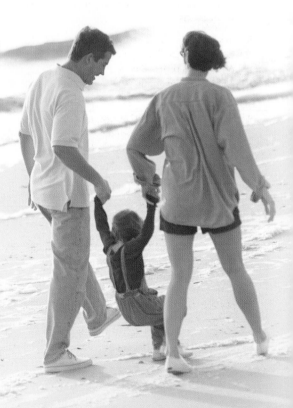

References

Chapter 1
Understanding your body

1   HFEA Guide to Infertility and Directory of Clinics. 2005–2006. Human Fertilisation and Embryology Authority.

2   Beus, T (2001). The menstrual cycle. Women's Health.

3   Knight, J. (1996) Diagrams of the menstrual cycle. http://www.fertilityuk.org/nfps20.html. Accessed in August 2005.

4   Paavonen, J. (2004). Sexually transmitted chlamydial infections and subfertility. *International Congress Series*. Vol 1266, 277-286.

5   Franks, S. (2005). Polycystic Ovary Syndrome and Subfertility. www.child.org.uk. Accessed August 2005.

6   Gilling-Smith, C. & Franks, S. (1993). Polycystic Ovary Syndrome. Medical Review 2, 15-32.

7   Endometriosis Society. (2005). What is endometriosis? www.endo.org.uk. Accessed in August 2005.

8   Swan, S.H., Elkin, E.P. and Fenster, L. 2000. The Question of Declining Sperm Density Revisited: An Analysis of 101 Studies Published 1934–1996. Environmental Health Perspective 108: 961-966.

9   Abell, A., Ernst, E., and Bonde, J.P. (1994). High sperm density among members of organic farmers' association. *Lancet* 343:1498.

10 Dawson, E.B., Harris, W.A. and Powell, L.C. (1990). Relationship between ascorbic acid and male fertility. In: Aspects of Some Vitamins, Minerals and Enzymes in Health and Disease. *World Rev Nutr Diet* 62:1-26 [review].

11 Rolf, C., Cooper, T.G. *et al* (1999). Antioxidant treatment of patients with asthenozoospermia or moderate oligoasthenozoospermia with high-dose vitamin C and vitamin E: a randomized, placebo-controlled, double-blind study. *Hum Reprod* 14: 1028-33.

12 Kynaston, H.G., Lewis-Jones, D.I. *et al* (1988). Changes in seminal quality following oral zinc therapy. *Andrologia*; 20:21-2.

13 De Aloysio, D., Mantuano, R. *et al* (1982). The clinical use of arginine aspartate in male infertility. *Acta Eur Fertil*; 13:133-67.

14 Sandler, B., Faragher, B. (1984). Treatment of oligospermia with vitamin B12. *Infertility*; 7:133-8.

15 Bayer, R. (1960). Treatment of infertility with vitamin E. *Int J Fertil*; 5:70-8.

16 Glenville, M. Natural Solutions to Infertility (2000). Piatkus Books. London.

17 Edmond, C.O. Edi-Osagie, M.D. *et al* Characterizing the endometrium in unexplained and tubal factor infertility: A multiparametric investigation.

18 Age and infertility – Figure 1: abstracted from National Bureau of Health Statistics, (2000). Figure 2: Gindoff and Jewelweicz, *Fertil Steril* 46:989, 1986. Figure 3: Munne S, Cohen J. *Hum Reprod* Update 4: 842, 1998.

19 About pregnancy loss (2005). The Miscarriage association. http://www.miscarriageassociation.org.uk. Accessed in August 2005.

20 Ward, N. Foresight 1990–1993 Study of Pre-conceptual Care and Pregnancy Outcome. *Journal of Nutritional & Environmental Medicine* (1995) 5, 205-208.

21 Lapane, K.L., Zierler, S. *et al* (1995). Is a history of depressive symptoms associated with an increased risk of infertility in women? *Psychosomatic Medicine* 1995 vol 57.

22 Green, B.B., Weiss, N.S., and Daling, J.R. (1988). Risk of ovulatory infertility in relation to body weight. *Fertility and Sterility* 50:5.

23 Grodstein, F., Goldman, M.B., and Cramer, D.W. (1994). Body Mass Index and Ovulatory Infertility. *Epidemiology* 5:2

24 Drs Larry Dulgisz, Michael Brahcs, Yale (1990). Coffee decreases fertility health 0. University school of medicine epidemological reviews vol 14:83.

25 Jelovsek, F.R., MD. Lifestyle Choices and Female Infertility http://www.wdxcyber.com/ninfer06.htm. Accessed September 2005.

26 American Society for Reproductive Medicine (2003). Smoking and Infertility. http://www.asrm.org/Patients/FactSheets/smoking.pdf. Accessed in September 2005.

27 Barnes, B. and Bradley, S.G. (1990). Planning for a Healthy Baby. Vermillion. London.

Chapter 2
Fertility testing

1 Roberts, J.E., Spandorfer, S. *et al* (2005). Taking a basal follicle-stimulating hormone history is essential before initiating in vitro fertilization. *Fertility and Sterility*; 83(1), 37-41.

2 Dana, M.D. and Naz, R.K. (1995). Infertility due to antisperm antibodies. *Urology* 46(4), 591-602.

3 Van Voorhis, B.J. and Stovall, D.W. (1997). Auto-antibodies and infertility: a review of the literature. *Journal of Reproductive Immunology* 33(3), 239-256.

4 www.labtestsonline.org.uk. Accessed in July 2005.

5 Basal Body Temperature charts. http://www.fertility.com. Accessed in July 2005.

6 Ward, N. (1995). Foresight 1990–1993 Study of Pre-conceptual Care and Pregnancy Outcome. *Journal of Nutritional & Environmental Medicine*; 5, 205-208.

7 Ohl, D.A. and Menge, A.C. (1996). Assessment of sperm functional and clinical aspects of sperm function. *Frontiers in Bioscience* 1, e96-108.

Chapter 3
Treatments

1 Barnes, B. and Bradley, S.G. (1990). Planning for a Healthy Baby. Vermillion. London

2 Miller, L, 'Is the answer at your feet?', *Daily Express,* Jan 29 2001.

3 Bradford, N. (2000). Encyclopedia of Complementary Health. Hamlyn. London (60-66).

4 Garner, C. 'Is your mind stopping you conceiving?', *Daily Express,* Jan 29 2001.

5 Manson, L., 'Baby Talk', *Sunday Times,* July 19 1998.

6 Propping, D. and Katzorke, T. (1987). Treatment of corpus luteum insufficiency. *Zeitschr Allgemeinmedizin*; 63:932-3

7 Acupuncture. http://www.betterhealth.vic.gov.au. Accessed in September 2005.

8 Billings, J.J. (2000). The Ovulation Method: Natural Family Planning. The Liturgical Press. Minnesota.

9 Huang, H.Y., Lee, C.L. *et al.* (1996). The impact of the total motile sperm count on the success of intrauterine insemination with husband's spermatozoa. *J Assist Reprod Genet* 13:1, 56-63.

10 Van Voorhis, B.J., Barnett, M. *et al.* Effect of the total motile sperm count on the efficacy and cost-effectiveness of intrauterine insemination and in vitro fertilization. Department of Obstetrics & Gynecology, University of Iowa College of Medicine, *Fertil Steril* 2001 Apr; 75(4):661-8.

11 Campana, A., Sakkas D. *et al.* (1996). Intrauterine insemination: evaluation of the results according to the woman's age, sperm quality, total sperm count per insemination and life table analysis. *Hum Reprod* 11(4):732-6.

Useful addresses

British Infertility Counsellors Association
69 Division Street
SHEFFIELD
South Yorkshire S4 1GE
Tel: 0114 263 1448
www.bica.net

The National Infertility Network
(INUK)
Charter House
43 St Leonards Road
Bexhill-on-Sea
East Sussex TN40 1JA
Tel: 08701 1888088
www.infertilitynetworkuk.com

COTS (Childlessness Overcome Through Surrogacy)
Lairg
Sutherland
IV27 4EF
Tel: 01549 402777
www.surrogacy.org.uk

Foresight Association
The Association for Promotion of Pre-Conception Care
178 Hawthorn Road
Bognor Regis
West Sussex PO21 2UY
Tel: 01243 868001
www.foresight-preconception.org.uk

Human Fertilisation & Embryology Authority (HFEA)
21 Bloomsbury Street
London
WC1B 3HF
Tel: 020 7291 8200
www.hfea.gov.uk

More to Life
Charter House
43 St Leonards Road
Bexhill-on-Sea
East Sussex TN40 1JA
Tel: 08701 1888088
www.infertilitynetworkuk.com

Multiple Birth Foundation
Queen Charlotte's & Chelsea Hospital
Goldhawk Road
London W6 0XG
Tel: 020 8383 3519
www.multiplebirths.org.uk

National Institute of Medical Herbalists
Elm House
54 Mary Arches Street
Exeter EX4 3BA
Tel: 01392 426022
www.nimh.org.uk

The British Complementary Medicine Association
PO Box 5122
Bournemouth BH8 0WG
Tel: 0845 345 5977
www.bcma.co.uk

The British Acupuncture Council
63 Jeddo Road
London W12 9HQ
Tel: 020 8735 0400
www.acupuncture.org.uk

The National Endometriosis Society
50 Westminster Palace Gardens
Artillery Row
London
SW1P 1RR
Tel:020 7222 2781
www.endo.org.uk

The Miscarriage Association
Clayton Hospital
Northgate
Wakefield
West Yorkshire WF1 3JS
Tel: 01924 200799
www.miscarriageassociation.org.uk

Verity (PCOS)
Unit AS20.01
The Aberdeen Centre
22-24 Highbury Grove
London N5 2EA
www.verity-pcos.org.uk

Useful websites:
www.babycentre.co.uk
www.fertilityfriends.co.uk

www.3stepstofertility.co.uk

This website was set up to give you the opportunity to keep abreast of the latest developments relating to infertility and allow you to meet other people who are trying to conceive a baby. You can contact people directly or just read their stories; your involvement is entirely up to you! In addition, you will find details on treatments, contact information and real stories from women who have successfully conceived a baby following the advice in this book. If you have a question or need advice, you can email Marina Nicholas, who is more than happy to answer your query. Visit the website today!

Index

Acupuncture 26, 44, 99, 103–7
Adoption 153, 154
Age
  and fertility 37, 41, 84
  and stillbirth 43
Alcohol and fertility 36, 48, 87
Amniocentesis 43
Anovulatory cycle 100
Asherman's syndrome 33
Assisted hatching (AH) 135, 136
Assisted reproductive
  technologies (ART) 39, 114
Autoimmune testing 71

Basal body temperature (BBT) 16,
  24, 74
Bicornate uterus 33
Billings method 99
Body mass index (BMI) 45, 46, 87

Caffeine 47, 87
Carbohydrates 88
Cervical mucus 15, 21, 99–100
Cervix 13
Chlamydia 21, 22, 37
Clinics, choosing 114–17
Cocaine 48
Cognitive behavioural therapy
  113
Complementary fertility tests 80
Complementary treatments 86
  see also acupuncture;
  herbal medicine;
  hypnotherapy; reflexology
COTS (Childlessness Overcome
  Through Surrogacy) 153
Counselling 52, 139
Cycle monitoring 130

Depression 49, 52, 148
Detox, 3-day 96
Detoxification 95
  foods that assist 51
Diabetes and older mothers 43

Diet
  and nutrition 86
  and PCOS 26
  pre-conception 87, 98
  whole food and infertility 40
Dilation and curettage (D&C) 33
Down's syndrome 43, 44, 48, 84

Ectopic pregnancy 13, 21, 23, 39,
  56
  causes and treatment 59
Egg
  collection 133
  donation 44, 141
  production and age 41–2
Embryo
  developing 136
  donation 141
  transfer 137
Emotional support 148
Endometrial biopsy 79
Endometriosis 20, 29–30, 59, 89,
  93
Endometrium 13
Environmental toxins 50
Essential Fatty Acids (EFAs) 89, 92
Exercise and PCOS 26

Fallopian tubes 13
  problems 20–23
Fats 89
Female sex hormones 13
Female sex organs 13
Fertilisation 19
Fertility
  and women's age 27
  drugs 131
  drugs, side effects 60
  testing 68, 130
  tests for men 72–3
  tests for women 74–9
  treatments 85 see also assisted
  reproductive technologies
Fetal abnormalities and age 43
Fetal Alcohol Syndrome (FAS) 48

Fibre 89
Fibroids 31–2, 59, 89, 93
Folic acid 90, 92
Follicle stimulating hormone
  (FSH) 14, 24–7, 41, 73, 77, 132
Follicular phase (menstrual cycle)
  15
Food preparation 89
Foresight
  Organisation/Programme 36,
  40, 80, 86, 87

Genetic disorders 71
Genital tract infections 21
GIFT (Gamete Intrafallopian
  Transfer) 140
Gonorrhoea 21, 22, 37

Hair mineral analysis (HMA) 36,
  81, 86–7
Herbal medicine 107–10
  and PCOS 26
Herbicides see toxins
Heroin 48
Hormonal imbalances 29
Hormone
  replacement therapy (HRT) 29
  tests for men 73
  tests for women 77
Human Fertilisation and
  Embryology Authority (HFEA)
  114, 120, 121, 123
Hypnotherapy 110–13
Hysterectomy 31, 32
Hysterosalpingogram (HSG) 23,
  32, 78
Hysteroscopy 32, 79, 130

Immune screening 130
Implantation 19
In vitro fertilisation (IVF) 23, 38,
  44, 114, 120, 123–39
  cycle diary 142–5
  process 128–9

Infertility
  couple factors 39–40
  female factors 20
  male factors 33
Insulin 24
Insulin Resistance Syndrome 46
Intracytoplasmic injection (ICSI) 33, 38, 114, 120, 134, 136
Intrauterine adhesions 33
Intrauterine insemination (IUI) 27, 44, 122

Klinefelters syndrome 37

Laparoscopy 23, 31, 79
Live birth rate data 118, 120
Losing weight 45
Low-birth-weight babies 43
Luteal phase (menstrual cycle) 15
Luteinising hormone (LH) 15, 24, 73, 77, 100

Male infertility 37
Male sex hormone 17
Male sex organs 17
Malformations of the uterus 33
Marijuana 48
Menstrual cycle 14, 100
Micromanipulation techniques 134–5
Mind-body therapy 52, 110
Minerals
  essential 91
  sources of 93
Miscarriage 39, 41, 42, 44, 45, 56–9, 86
Multiple births 123
Myomectomy 32

Obesity and fertility 45
Oestradiol (E2) 77
Oestrogen 13, 15, 89, 93
  and fibroids 31
Organic food 40, 50, 87
Ovarian hyperstimulation syndrome (OHSS) 39, 44, 56, 60–61, 122
Ovarian reserve 27, 41–2, 43
Ovarian stimulation 132

Ovaries 13
Overweight 24
Ovulation 15
  induction (OI) 121
  method 99, 100
  predictor kits 77, 78
  problems 20, 23, 24
  signs of 15
  test kit 100

Pelvic inflammatory disease (PID) 20–21, 59
Penis 17
Pesticides see toxins
Polycystic ovarian syndrome (PCOS) 23, 24, 26, 46, 89, 93, 99, 122
Polyps 32
Pre-conception plan 94–9
Pre-eclampsia 45
Pregnancy tests 19
Pre-implantation genetic diagnosis (PGD) 135
Premature menopause 29
Premature ovarian failure (POF) 29
Progesterone 13, 15, 77
Prolactin 29, 73, 77
Prostate gland 17
Proteins 88
Psychological factors and fertility 49

Recreational drugs 48, 87
Reflexology 26, 44, 99, 101–3
Relaxation 52
Retrograde menstruation 30
Rhesus (Rh) test 76
Rubella (German measles) 76

Secondary infertility 55
Septate uterus 33
Sexually transmitted diseases (STDs) 21, 22
  and sperm production 33
  tests for 70
Smoking 87
  effect on sperm 36
  effect on women 47–8

Sperm
  count 33–4, 72, 89
  donation 141
  health, nutritional and environmental factors 36
  motility 72
  production 17–19, 33–4, 35, 36
  surgical aspiration of 135
  survival time 15, 99
Spina bifida 90
Stress 39, 49
Support groups 149
Surrogacy 153
Syphilis 22

Testicles 17
  see also sperm production
Testing, fertility 68
Testosterone 17, 34, 73
Thrush 22
Toxins 80, 87
  environmental 50
Traditional Chinese Medicine (TCM) 107
Tubal disease 20–23

Ultrasound 78
Uterine fibroids 31–2
Uterine polyp 32
Uterine problems 20
Uterus 13
  malformed 33

Varicocele 34
Vitamins 86
  essential 90
  for sperm production 35–6
  sources of 92
  supplementation 98
Vitex 108

Water intake 90
Website support 52
Weight
  and fertility 45
  losing 45

ZIFT (Zygote Intrafallopian Transfer) 140

Acknowledgements

I would like to thank Simon, my husband, for his incredible love and support throughout this journey; for believing that we could overcome the odds, for never giving up hope and for encouraging me to write this book. You are my rock that has kept me sane throughout this whole roller coaster ride!

A big thank you to my Mum who has helped me get through the last seven years emotionally and physically. She truly is one of the world's greatest carers and has put me on the road to recovery after every one of my operations.

Thanks to my friends and family for their compassion and understanding over the years; for putting up with my mad moments and pulling me out of the depths of despair. You have been a tremendous support and have kept me motivated to carry on trying for a baby.

I would like to thank the practitioners whom I have met along the way and who helped me achieve my dream of having a baby. Mr Taranissi, Julie, Angela and the rest of the team at the ARGC clinic for their outstanding treatment and dedication. I have never seen a team of people work so hard, be so focused and commit so much time to helping couples achieve their

dream. Laura Gerrard, my reflexologist for her constant encouragement over the last five years and always knowing what to do to make me feel better. Elizabeth Muir, my hypnotherapist for making me realise that I can have a baby if I believe in myself and helping eradicate years of negative thoughts. Daniel Elliott for his valuable contribution on acupuncture and herbal medicine. Belinda Barnes and the team at Foresight for the hair analysis results that started us on the road to improving our diet and health.

Special thanks to our friend Jane Whittaker who spent numerous hours reading the first chapter and lending her valuable medical expertise to the book. To Lauren Johnston who encouraged me to write to a publisher with the idea for this book and gave me the details of Carroll & Brown. To Amy Carroll, my editor, for believing in my idea and giving me the chance to help other infertile couples though this book.

Finally, I would like to thank the special women who have contributed their own personal stories so that others can be inspired and encouraged by their success. I am extremely grateful to you all for taking the time to recount your stories and for making this book real.

Carroll & Brown would like to thank:
Designer Laura de Grasse
Illustrations Denise Brown
Production Director Karol Davies
IT Management Paul Stradling
Picture Researcher Sandra Schneider

Picture credits
Front jacket Photolibrary
Back jacket (right), pages 3, 5, 82 Dragan Mikki
Page 50 (left) Harvey Pincis/SPL
Page 51 (bottom) Dave Reede/Agstock/SPL
Page 60–61 GE Healthcare
Page 69 Punchstock/PhotoAlto
Page 73 (bottom) Pasquale Sorrentino/SPL
Page 78 Du Cane Medical Centre Ltd/SPL
Page 79 John Greim/SPL
Page 101 Michelangelo Gratton/SPL
Page 103 Photolibrary
Page 127 Punchstock/Comstock
Page 128 (top left) Mauro Fermariello/SPL; (top right) John McLean /SPL; (bottom left) Mauro Fermariello/SPL; (bottom right) Hank Morgan/SPL
Page 129 (top left) Hank Morgan/SPL; (top right) Andy Walker, Midland Fertility Services/SPL; (bottom left) Alexander Tsiaras/SPL; (bottom right), John McLean/SPL
Page 134 Zephyr/SPL
Page 135 (top) Andy Walker, Midland Fertility Services/SPL; (bottom) Pascal Goetgheluck/SPL